VOICES OF CONCERN

"Any patient being transported by helicopter is the sickest of the sick. It's just you and that other nurse up there running the show, monitoring the patient's status, radioing ahead to the hospital telling them what you've got and what you'll need on arrival. And delivering what care you can."

"Letting go doesn't mean that if you lose a patient, if a patient dies, that you don't grieve for that person. You do. I've grieved for every patient I've lost."

"Then there's the Friday night melee when, say, during a code, a family gets into a brawl in the ER, trying to kill each other as their way of expressing grief. It can get so damn crazy some nights."

"She looked into my eyes for the full twenty minutes it took her to die. She held my hand. And I wasn't allowed to do anything."

"You just never know. You try to learn as much as you can, to do the best job you can. But you just never know."

NURSES

The Human Touch

Michael Brown, R.N.

IVY BOOKS • NEW YORK

Ivy Books
Published by Ballantine Books
Copyright © 1992 by Michael Brown

Library of Congress Catalog Card Number: 91-92407

ISBN 0-8041-0800-5

Manufactured in the United States of America

First Edition: July 1992

Cover photos by Robert Llewellyn/Superstock

CONTENTS

ACKNOWLEDGMENTS

This book could not have been written without the help of many people. Foremost, I am indebted to all the nurses who took the time to share their insights and experiences with me. While not everyone is represented in the text, each nurse I interviewed helped extend my understanding of our profession, for which I am profoundly grateful. I'd like to take this space to acknowledge those nurses who requested to be identified by their full names: Donna Pffeifer, Kathleen Diamond, Barbara Siebelt, and Frank Bartholemew.

Several people were helpful with research, editorial advice, moral support, professional expertise, and reality testing. Nurses who assisted in this regard were Doris Jacobs, Debbie Mulgrew and the PCU and 2NE crews, Mary Beth Kenny, Doris Keyser, Melva Dill, Paula Goldberg, Kathleen Marion and, in a clutch situation, Mary Beth Hare. The support and direction of Maureen Faulkner were incalculably valuable. Doctors who lent a hand included Mark Novitsky, Anne Tyson, Mike Glackin, David Mozley, and everyone in Crisis. Regards also to my two favorite social workers, Gwen James and Linda Johnson. Civilian input came from Donald Hetz, Alan Doelp, Kathleen Platt Clark, Lyn Watner, and Mike Himowitz. I am particularly obliged to Jim Wooton, Ron Shapiro, Lyn Scholz, and Leslie Walker.

Much appreciation is due my agent, Dominick Abel, who immediately grasped the possibility of a book and remained committed to it even during difficult times. Barbara Dicks, my editor at Fawcett, brought fresh eyes and a deft hand to editing the manuscript.

My gratitude to Val and George Musat, Steve White, Dorene Suarez, Connie Russell, Betty Morgan, and Matt Bokar. All generously supplied me with lodgings allowing me access to areas of the country to which I might not otherwise have been able to travel.

Many thanks to my parents, Edward and Dorothy Brown, for everything and more, and to Guy and Eleanor Simmons, whose enthusiasm for this project never wavered.

Finally, to my wife, Melody Simmons, I can offer only inadequate praise. She encouraged this project from the start and remained enthusiastic even when it dragged on much longer than anticipated. When I became disheartened, she remained steadfast. She coached me through computer nightmares and tape transcriptions, deadline sweats and innumerable revisions. The honesty and zeal she brings to all endeavors is a constant inspiration. For her wisdom and love I am thankful beyond telling.

AUTHOR'S NOTE

In preparing this book, more than fifty practicing nurses and several RN-tracked students were interviewed about their experiences and opinions. The clinical experience of participants ranged from less than one to over thirty years in the field, spanning forty-one states and most nursing specialities.

This book combines descriptive narrative with first-person perspectives. In either format, the attitudes expressed are those of the nurses described. To convey the emotional impact of particular situations, dialogue has been augmented, characterizations broadened, and details added. All such embellishments are based upon common nursing situations encountered directly by me or related to me by nurses and other health professionals.

In an attempt to guarantee the confidentiality of any patients described and encourage ease of disclosure, participants were informed that as far as possible, no institutions or individuals named would be identified; in most instances not even the city or state where they currently practice is mentioned. Obviously, all patient names and personal characteristics are fictitious.

Each nurse was given a choice of how to be identified—full name, first name, or pseudonym—depending upon the degree of confidentiality with which she or he felt most comfortable. The majority wished to be described by first names only, and this became the standard adopted throughout. (Pseudonyms were used upon request. For nurses with the same first name, spelling variations are employed to distinguish individuals when possible.)

Because health care is rife with technical jargon, abbreviations, acronyms, and slang, brief explanations are included within the text in order to avoid frequent reference to a glossary. I hope such insertions do not prove too distracting.

Finally, because nurses are present in so many areas of health care delivery, education, and research, decisions related to space constraints had to be made. It was my choice to place the greatest emphasis on those who have direct patient contact in hospital settings, where the majority practice. This was not meant to slight any other nurses, all of whom pride themselves upon being professional RNs.

INTRODUCTION

News reports about the crisis in health care have become commonplace. In less than a decade, the face of the entire industry has changed. Numerous social and political forces—Reaganomics; an explosion in technological advances, epidemics in drug abuse, homelessness and communicable diseases, growing numbers of aging patients, and rising physician fees at odds with tightening insurance restrictions—arrived like overlapping waves, battering the system from within and without.

A major component of the health care crisis is the nationwide shortage of registered nurses. Headlines have described the shortage as "pervasive" and "epidemic," its "dire effects" touching every aspect of health care. In December 1988, a federal panel appointed to investigate the problem by Otis Bowen, then secretary of Health and Human Services, issued its first report characterizing the shortage as "of significant magnitude" and concluded that it was starting to "erode the quality of health care as well as access to services." The most dramatic indications of the shortage have been reports of intensive care unit and emergency room closings, respective symbols of medicine's most high-tech and essential services.

At the beginning of the 1990s, nationwide estimates of the number of vacancies for positions requiring a registered nurse range from 100,000 to 300,000 and are expected to double by the end of the decade. In January 1991, the *American Journal of Nursing* (AJN) reported that of 999 nursing homes surveyed by the American Nurses' Association (ANA), nearly one-fifth of RN positions went unfilled. In its March '91 issue, the AJN reported instances of staff shortages compromising care and endangering lives in a geriatric psych unit in Virginia and a Los Angeles neonatal intensive care unit. While there are more registered nurses today than ever before—their numbers rising past the two million mark in 1988—several trends, both in health care and the larger culture, have coalesced to create current conditions.

The Bowen Report panel had deduced that the nursing shortage was "primarily the result of an increase in demand, as opposed to a contraction in supply." Increasing numbers of AIDS victims, drug-related hospital admissions, and the elderly have translated directly into a need for nurses. In March '91, *The New York Times* reported that the elderly population is growing at a rate double that of the population in general. "Moreover, the elderly population itself is aging, with a larger proportion consisting of people over seventy-five years old, who require more care than those sixty-five to seventy-five." In hospitals, where 70 percent of working nurses are employed, the explosion of technological developments has increased the need for highly skilled and knowledgeable personnel to manage the machinery that sustains life. That has translated into a need for more RNs, often by regulatory statute.

Probably the single-most significant event impacting upon health care in the United States in the last decade was the restructuring of the entire method of payment for services delivered to the public. Medicare prospective pricing for services—commonly referred to as DRGs (diagnostic-related groups)—originated as part of a broad legislative package with Congressional passage of the Social Security Amendments of 1983. This legislation was the result of years of effort to control skyrocketing health expenditures initiated in the 1960s with the creation of Medicare and Medicaid, which expanded health coverage to millions of previously unserved citizens.

In pre-DRG days, health providers were reimbursed retrospectively for each dollar spent on patient care. Under the new plan, Medicare—with other health insurers following suit—pays for services on the basis of pre-established "average" rates for diagnostic-related groups of illnesses. Put simply, DRGs mean that if a patient is admitted to a hospital for an ailment—which statistics show should, on average, require three days of care at a cost of $2,000—then that amount of money is given as a flat fee. The built-in incentive is to treat and discharge patients as quickly as possible because the dollar difference between the projected cost and the actual cost is retained and a profit made. However, if the patient is unable to be discharged in the average time, the hospital loses revenue.

A second major outgrowth of DRGs was the tightening of hospital-admission criteria, requiring more severe degrees of illness or impairment to gain entry, thus increasing the need for more intensive nursing care.

Initially, most health care analysts did not foresee how intimately DRGs and hospital nursing services would be bound together. In 1983, which saw the largest increase in nursing school enrollment in twenty years, there was a perceived RN market glut. Many hospital administrators, foreseeing potential financial shortfalls as a consequence of DRGs, cut back on nursing positions.

Over the eighteen months it took for that to evolve into a nursing shortage—when administrators finally realized that the impact of DRGs was to *in*crease the patient acuity level (degree of illness) and therefore the demand for more nurses—those nurses had gone into other areas.

At the very time when more nurses were needed in hospitals, RNs were also being siphoned away by other modes of health care delivery. Nurses traditionally have worked outside hospitals in areas such as public health—visiting home nurses, school nurses—private industry, the armed services, and higher education. The past fifteen years have witnessed the emergence of other employment possibilities. HMOs, PHPs, freestanding clinics, "doc in the box" walk-in centers, and private-practice models frequently require the presence of RNs to attain licensure. There has also been a sharp increase in the numbers of

nurses receiving master's and doctoral degrees allowing them to
move into more independent practice spheres. Nurses are also
being enticed into other fields—pharmaceutical sales, computers, real estate, entrepreneurial endeavors—where their keen or-
ganizational skills are substantially rewarded.

Simultaneously, cultural directions developed that strike at
the heart of the profession. At a time when women have far
greater options in career selection—doctor, astronaut, Supreme
Court justice—the "female profession" of nursing has fallen
into disfavor. Its image as a passive, peripheral vocation, a
"support" to the "important work" of physicians, holds little
allure for women who wish to exercise mastery over their careers. There is a common perception that nurses are undercom-
pensated for jobs requiring imposing physical labor and
psychological stress. In 1987, for the first time, more incoming
female college freshmen declared medicine over nursing as their
intended major.

Anna, an adult family nurse practitioner with over fifteen years
in practice, summed it up:

"I don't know what is going to happen. They can't keep
nurses, and they're not making as many as they used to.
Women have other options in society, and they are exercising
them. There's more money to be made elsewhere. There's
more dignity to be had. There are more intellectually stimu-
lating and less physically demanding jobs out there. There are
places you can go to work looking good and smelling good,
and come home the same way with more energy left over and
more money to spend enjoying it."

Against this tide, hospitals are scrambling to fill positions. Salaries have increased across the board. The October 1991 issue
of *RN Magazine* reported a survey that touted nursing salaries
as having risen 17 percent in two years, contrasted with an 11
percent hike in the cost of living. Numerous inducements are
being employed to recruit new nurses and retain those with ex-

perience: sign-on bonuses of several thousand dollars, relocation allowances, subsidized housing, educational benefits expanded to include family members, bounties to staff nurses who
recruit friends, and merit incentives. In 1990 a new hospital in
the University of Texas system inaugurated a nine-month,
schoolteacher-mode, work-year schedule for staff RNs.

Nursing recruiters travel around the country and as far away
as Canada, Ireland, and the Philippines to lure nurses to better-
paying, stateside employment. But not without problems.
Fifteen percent of New York City's RNs are foreign-nursing
graduates. In 1988, a desperate Veterans Administration sparked
controversy when it openly recruited nurses from Puerto Rico,
waiving the requirement that they pass state nursing exams demanded of stateside nurses for licensure and calling into question the quality of care being afforded patients in VA hospitals.

Many observers view such "solutions" as makeshift measures, Band-Aids applied to a hemorrhage.

Within the work force, there are issues that predate Florence
Nightingale but continue to cause resentment: interference from
the dominant medical community, the amount and method of
compensation for services, hospital administrations that give
only lip service to the notion of nurses defining the parameters
of their own practice. The desire to be accorded respect and
authority commensurate with the responsibility carried by each
nurse is keenly felt and continues to go largely unfulfilled.

Many seasoned RNs, having witnessed shortage scares before, scoff at hospital promos huckstering nursing care in the
newly competitive health care environment: "Our nurses offer
the personal touch. . . ." "When you reach out for someone in
the middle of the night, our nurses are there."

"It's funny," a Philadelphia nurse with eighteen years' experience observed. "Nobody gave a damn about us until we
started to disappear."

1

"Running the Show"

Extended Scope

Fifteen hundred feet and climbing, the chopper cruised eastward toward the coast, casting its shadow across the North Carolina countryside. The pilot hailed the flight-control tower, identifying his call numbers and purpose—"lifeguard mission, Medevac"—seeking emergency permission to cross crowded airspace. It was often necessary to traverse airfields, civilian and military, day and night. Access was rarely denied.

Behind him in the cabin, Cindy and her flight-nurse partner, Pam, sat at alert, faces to their windows, microphones in hand. They scanned for potential hazards, extra eyes for the pilot. During missions, every member of the team worked to safeguard the helicopter and bring it in.

"Aircraft, three o'clock," Cindy said calmly. "No factor . . ." Nothing to indicate danger.

Quite often it *was* a factor.

Crossing airfields was the only time Cindy favored night flight, since planes are easier to spot. They listened to the radio squawk for any further word on their mission as well as weather broadcasts and air traffic patterns. Despite the close quarters within the Bell Long Ranger cabin, crowded with advanced life support equipment, she preferred it to small fixed-wing planes. There was better visibility than she'd experienced in Pipers and Apaches, and the ride was smoother.

Twenty minutes earlier, when Cindy's belt beeper sounded, she'd experienced the semi-ready, semi-dread catecholamine surge that accompanied each flight. The thrill of the focused moment. People in aviation tend to work well under pressure, crisis-control types who savor the stress. Trauma demands an immediate response. Treatment is a race against time, an attempt to interrupt the inevitable shock process triggered by an "insult to the system." Untreated, shock becomes irreversible, resulting in stagnant blood flow, multiple organ failure, and death.

Only a sketchy outline of the mission had been radioed ahead. Larry P., a thirty-eight-year-old Caucasian male driver of a logging truck, was the sole victim of a collision; he'd fallen asleep at the wheel and been ejected by the impact, suffering near-fatal head injuries. Transported by ambulance to an outlying community hospital, he'd been judged too drastically impaired to receive adequate treatment there.

Cindy began her mental preparations, shaking out an initial list of priorities, running potential complications through her head. The soles of her high-top safety boots tapped in anticipation. They were laced snugly for ankle support when hitting the ground, with steel-toed reinforcers for working around the broken glass and metal shards that litter accident sites.

Illuminating stripes ran down the sides of her flight suit so she could be seen in the dark. The flapped and zippered pockets bulged with devices essential in the field—hemastats, trauma scissors, tourniquets, bandages, tape, gloves. One side pocket was reserved for a supply of angiocaths, the first on-scene task usually being the starting of an IV. Her breast pocket held a "cheat book" with IV drip dosages, resuscitation fluid rates like the Parkland Formula for burn victims, and conversion tables for pediatric use, which could be flipped to in a hurry. While new to trauma fieldwork, Cindy had already learned to keep an extra O_1 wrench stashed away, indispensable for opening the portable oxygen canisters hauled to scenes, having experienced the icy frustration of one breaking during a damp night mission with no replacement available.

She'd also learned to stuff pockets with more personal items. Granola bars and trail mix provided quick energy on the days when there was no break in the action. Flying on an empty stomach left her terribly nauseous. Being "weathered in" for the night in airports taught her to carry a contact case and a small supply of eyewash as well as a comb and brush, toothbrush and paste.

"So I'm vain," she would shrug when teased by the flight crew. "I admit it."

Flight crews weigh in at the start of each shift. Before loading her pockets, Cindy weighed 128 pounds. Afterward, 136. There were days when her pant legs dragged on the ground.

With reddish hair and an easy, wry smile, Cindy resembles Carol Burnett. Standing close to five feet eight inches, she is muscular from regular workouts. Field missions demand a certain amount of physical exertion. Many flight programs around the country encourage a 180-pound lift limit, to prepare for lugging cumbersome equipment across awkward terrain, not to mention the deadweight of a body on a stretcher.

Air-ambulance programs exist in a variety of compositions. The field team consists of one pilot and either two nurses or two paramedics or a nurse/paramedic mix. The latter has become the industry norm, used in 86 percent of the over 150 hospital-based helicopter programs across the United States.

North Carolina employed only registered nurses. It gave Cindy a great deal of pride to be working in an area she considered on the cutting edge of her profession: to be a member of the National Flight Nurses Association and to be following in the footsteps of pioneers who struggled through years of controversy and cynicism when others in both fields, aviation and nursing, were insisting that flight nurses would never be used to their full potential.

Cindy treasured the transition from hospital nursing to fieldwork, embracing the increased autonomy and independence. In recent years, the scope of practice of nurses has broadened tremendously, extending to duties and responsibilities previously reserved for physicians. Nowhere is this more so than in an area like flight nursing. Cindy gladly accepted the challenge to all the knowledge and skill she had gained throughout her career, even when the responsibilities tied knots in her stomach.

"Any patient being transported by helicopter is the sickest of the sick. It's just you and that other nurse up there running the show, monitoring the patient's status, radioing ahead to the hospital telling them what you've got and what you'll need on arrival.

"You deliver what care you can. Of course, the ultimate rule is: *Do no further harm.*"

Essentially, two Medevac operating scenarios exist: Interhospital transfers and off-the-road (OTR) missions.

This flight was one of the former.

Hospitals have set helipads. Typically, before landing, the copter does a high-reconnaissance spin around, scanning for obstacles on deck. There have been dogs asleep on landing pads, trash lying about, and loose paint chips. Even stray pieces of paper that get sucked up by the prop wash into the intake valve, leaving crews stranded with a downed helicopter, a maintenance bill climbing into the thousands of dollars, and a deteriorating patient going nowhere.

In hospitals unschooled in the uses of helicopters, staff have greeted them pulling gurneys with unsecured mattresses—and if they really want to be nice, a few loose sheets slung over them—which have caused considerable damage. Hats, jewelry, even loose lab coats have been known to be sucked up by the pressure.

Cindy remained watchful as they set down, working the mike, and feeling the tension tug of her responsibilities on the ground about to begin.

"It's the patients who have cardiac problems or who are critically ill, inter-hospital transfers with a multitude of illness, who are the ones it's trickiest to transport. They're basically time bombs. It's a cramped environment, and you don't have the luxury of the diagnostic capabilities you'll have at the hospital.

"You have some equipment. You try to resuscitate and stabilize to the best of your ability. If you're lucky, you may be able to use a ventilator or a pulse oximiter or a CO_2 monitor. You can have fourteen lines hanging, and be monitoring hemodynamic pressure with a Life-stat blood-pressure cuff as well as a catheter inserted for cardiac monitoring.

"It's bad when somebody arrests, and you're trying to resuscitate while pulling out, maybe trying to intubate or start the first round of cardiac drugs. Maybe they're bleeding, maybe screaming. It can get very hectic very fast."

The other team members went to assess Mr. P. as Cindy flipped through his chart noting fluid replacement forms, flow sheets, and graphs while listening to a report from the ER nurse. The damage was pervasive. He'd been traveling at about seventy miles an hour when he rear ended another semitrailer. The hospital did not have the surgical capability to secure an airway.

When going into a critical care, inter-hospital transfer situation, it is the flight nurse's responsibility to integrate all information relating to the patient's treatment thus far—X rays, blood gases, vital signs, social history, etc. The patient may have been in that hospital anywhere from a few hours to several days or weeks, long enough for him to become too critically ill to be managed. One hopes everything relevant is charted. There is a saying about the amount of attendant paperwork: For every patient who enters the system, a tree dies.

In this instance it was brief, proportional to his stay. It seemed a clear-cut case, despite the multisystem trauma—bilaterally fractured femurs, head injuries, a pneumothorax (gas or air in the tissue that enfolds the lungs). Just package the patient and go.

Then Pam returned, ashen-faced.

"Cindy, this man is just too sick to move."

"He'll never make it," the pilot concurred.

Cindy followed them to his cubicle. She had been a nurse for eight years, her career beginning as an ER staff nurse after she graduated from a diploma school in Louisville, Kentucky. During the following years, she gained experience in critical care, surgical and in-hospital trauma nursing. Still, Mr. P.'s condition caused her to catch her breath. He had the worst facial trauma she had ever seen. There were no connecting bones left. He had goulash features—no nose, cheeks, or forehead where they should have been. If one side of his face were touched, the other would slide away. His neck was twice its normal size, looking like two footballs and prohibiting the securing of a surgical airway. He had subcutaneous emphysema. This means the skin is puffed up by gas or air trapped in the subcutaneous tissue. The slang for it is "Rice Crispies," because of the crackling sounds the gas makes.

Making matters truly awful, he was conscious, if barely able to whimper, following them with helpless eyes.

Yet, he was breathing.

"I leave it to you guys," the ER physician said amiably, understanding the dilemma. "This is what you do all the time. You need to decide what you can handle. All I can tell you is that there's nothing else we can do for him here. It's a shit situation for sure. I'll support you either way."

As senior flight nurse, Cindy had to make the decision to hold or run with it. The three of them ran through the options, agonizing over outcomes. She felt her pulse racing, perspiration rings starting to form. What to do? Did they leave this man in the hospital when the nearest ear, nose, and throat surgeon was forty-five minutes away? Did they dare to even lay him down and risk compromising his cervical spine, possibly losing what little airway remained?

"You have to examine your options, and sometimes you don't have any. I think every time a nurse goes on a mission like that, whether in the back of an ambulance or in aviation, you wonder, 'Am I doing everything I can? Am I as smart as I can be? Am I able to troubleshoot these problems as quickly and most therapeutically as I can?'

"You go through that, but you have a certain amount of confidence in yourself as well. Sometimes you just hold your breath, grit your teeth, and do it. That's why it's so important to maintain your skills, that you have constant continuing education. This is not the arena you want to be slipping and sliding in."

They ran with it.

Weather is never static and conditions change quickly. At lift-off, the day was clear, well within weather minimums. For daytime flights, the rule was eight hundred-and-two, meaning visibility of eight hundred feet cloud ceiling and two miles in circumference. (Nowadays, if a flight call comes in and the weather is bad, either in the departure area or at the destination, they won't fly. Twenty years ago, there existed a rodeo cowboy attitude of "we're out there to save lives no matter what!" There were accidents because of that attitude. Now nobody flies in weather that is not safe. Rescuers have to go by ground. It is unfortunate for that person hemorrhaging in an auto accident or that stabbing victim, but crews are not risked.)

They were cruising at altitude when they punched into fog. At first, those in the rear were unaware, crouched and kneeling on the floor, focused on infusing blood and monitoring air exchange.

Pam noticed it first in the sway of the IV fluids.

"Cindy," she whispered.

Then they felt it, ever so slightly, the helicopter tilting. They looked at each other, then out the windows. It was Cindy's first experience with fog. It was not a feeling she liked. It engulfed the craft. All they could see was milky white.

"Oh" was all she could say.

It is essential for a pilot in such circumstances to switch from flying by visual cues to reliance on his instrument panel. What he needs to be most concerned about is not becoming confused. Vertigo can easily overtake him. In this instance, the pilot immediately went to instruments despite some dizziness. He later told them, "It was like this little voice was on my shoulder going, 'Look out the window! Just look out the window!' " Instead, he got on the radio, making a swift recovery, talking to flight control, telling them his heading and requesting to be vectored around.

In the rear, it was difficult for Cindy not to transmit her fear to the patient. Like the pilot, she concentrated on technique, doing what she could.

"Punching into that fog became a metaphor for many situations in nursing. Later, that is, when I started breathing regularly again. You find yourself in a situation that can go sour in an instant, something you have little or no control over, uncertain of your direction or position, dependent upon the technology you employ and the skills of those you work with, demanding every ounce of attention and expertise you can muster to focus on what is essential and not be distracted by the tension of the moment, the crisis surrounding you."

Upon arrival, a team of two surgeons required over an hour of surgical intervention to secure an airway. (Eventually, Mr. P. recovered nicely, leaving the hospital after a month of rehab, with no lingering problems.) They caught up to Cindy doing her in-house rounds.

"We just can't believe that you folks brought him in! He had closed-casket written all over him."

"You guys don't know the half of it."

* * *

There are over eight million disabling accidents annually in the United States. Approximately one hundred thousand will end in death, about one every four minutes. That's one thousand injuries and eleven deaths each hour. Trauma ranks as the fourth highest cause of death in the U.S. and Canada, just behind heart disease, cancer, and strokes. For those in their thirties or younger, it is *the* leading cause. Over half are motor vehicle accidents, more each year than the entire body count of the Vietnam War. Alcohol is involved in more than 50 percent of these, whether during holiday periods or not. Saturday is the worst day, August the bloodiest month.

During an off-the-road (OTR) mission, accident victims are transported directly from the scene to the nearest facility that can treat the injuries. There is a combatlike tension when people are coming in, the team never certain what they'll find. It is necessary to remain acutely vigilant, searching for odd, outstretched tree limbs, uneven terrain, all those things that are difficult to see from the air.

"There's a wire on the left-hand side. . . ."

"Cyclone fence in the shadow of the tree . . ."

Speed is the priority in an OTR. "Load-and-go" is the phrase for it. The helicopter sets down and the loads are done "hot," with rotor blades turning. Trauma patients aren't going to benefit from lengthy intervention at the scene. The speediest route to a surgical suite is the best treatment.

"On-scene patients usually have a lot of nuts-and-bolts-type injuries—broken bones and holes that you plug up and airways to be addressed. These are the kind of patients that people like myself and other flight nurses and flight paramedics like to care for. We're like addicts, to a degree. We're like people who like fast food for immediate gratification. When you are able to turn someone back over to their family, somebody you've salvaged, and they turn to you and say, 'Thank you, you did a wonderful job . . .' it is very grand. You thrive on that."

When all goes smoothly, and the initial ground providers—be they state police or ambulance crews—have the patient packaged tight for takeoff, ground times can be as short as five minutes. Complicating factors frequently lengthen that time. And then, there are the rare times when chaos reigns, when there aren't enough supplies or manpower, when there isn't enough expertise to go around. . . .

Local police sent out a disaster call, the highest priority, for a school bus crash with multiple injuries. The helicopter team arrived as the first advanced life support group. As they touched down, crew members were stormed by police and volunteers, who literally ripped every piece of available equipment from their hands and raced back. There were seventeen injured children. Luckily, when they received the call, the team thought far enough ahead to load up with extra fluids, bandages, blankets, and equipment.

Still, it wasn't enough.

It became necessary to institute military triage, making judgments about which children could and could not be saved, separating according to severity of injury, jumping from child to child, trying to intubate and get an IV line started before going on to the next one and then the next. For everyone involved, it was pure horror.

"Lives were saved, but it was a real helpless feeling. Those of us in emergency medicine sort of see ourselves as: *Save all life, end all pain.* When you can't see that patient through, when you've just got to go from starting an airway to dressing a gross hemorrhage to passing over that person with a bone sticking out of their leg, it chills you. Decisions had to be made between children who were in cardiac arrest versus children who had not arrested, but were profusely bleeding. Who to transport out first?

"It's emotionally wracking if you have any compassion at all. But that's triage; you want to do the most you can for the largest amount instead of the few. Another helicopter company arrived and were transporting kids out as quickly as possible. But it wasn't quick enough.

"The hours in that day just went on and on and on."

Cindy was working in a trauma center near Tampa, Florida, when she became aware of a program for Mobile Intensive Care Nurses in North Carolina. Because staffing levels for rural emergency departments were skeletal, they employed RNs to provide radio orders for emergency medical service (EMS) units. Similar systems exist in parts of California, Arkansas, and other states as well. For several years, she'd had the growing desire to be involved in Medevac work, coming to feel she would be unable to put closure on the "hands-on" part of her nursing career unless she became a flight nurse.

She contacted North Carolina and found that the people there were devoted to the concept of the emergency department nurse as a professional. She was single and unattached, living in fairly plush surroundings along the Gulf Coast, but was willing to do whatever it took to gain a new piece of career experience. The job offer in Chapel Hill requested that she begin in two weeks. It meant liquidating and leaving very quickly.

"For me, that was appropriate. I wasn't in the air, but it was a stepping-stone to gain the type of education that's necessary for a flight nurse."

It turned out to be exactly the right decision. It wasn't long afterward, while attending a course on basic trauma life support, that a man who was one of the moving forces in the local trauma community leaned over her shoulder during a lecture and whispered, "Do you like to fly?"

"Sure," she replied. "Where are we going?"

"Greenville . . . We're going to set up a new flight group there. I'd like you to come by in two weeks and put in an application."

"Okay," she said matter-of-factly while thinking, Wow, this is really happening!

A month later, she had the job.

Other team members came from across the country, recruited specifically for the program. There were seven other nurses and a medical director—none of whom had previous flight experience—and pilots, mechanics, and secretaries. The country was new to everyone. It was the second program set up in the state, covering thirty-four rural counties, including the coastal area and outer banks.

The hours were brutal. Shifts were twelve hours long and rotated from a month of days to a month of nights. They worked three days on, two days off, then reversed it. Still, Cindy loved it. There was exhilaration in laying the groundwork for a new system, setting up philosophies and goals, quality assurance and continuing-education seminars. Everyone, every piece of it, worked collaboratively, learning to respect each other's skills and areas of expertise. After her experience in the fog, witnessing the pilot's recovery, she developed a great deal of confidence in the pilots she flew with.

Being located in a small community, they became a very close-knit group, receiving much direct feedback from those they served. It was not uncommon for people in the area to write notes in the local paper: *Thanks to the flight team*, ever careful to recall the names of the nurses. *You saved my son's life*.

Around the time that Cindy arrived, there was much discussion about regionalizing the entire system, strategically stationing five flight groups around the state. As in many other areas that have flirted with regionalization, the plans became bogged down in political skirmishes and financial realities. It can be quite an expensive undertaking; for example, the state of Maryland—the only place in the United States where there is an integrated statewide system—spent $41 million in 1989 to acquire nine state-of-the-art trauma helicopters.

Because the state did not allocate funds, private hospitals moved into the patient retrieval business. Despite the concern that many patients who are victims of blunt and penetrating trauma—"gun-and-knife-club members"—are oftentimes underinsured, if insured at all, hospitals soon found it was an image boost as well as a financial incentive to become designated a "trauma center." Trauma incidents often involve multiple injuries to multiple victims who commonly engage the services of several hospital departments, the reimbursement ripple extending throughout the system.

The enhancement in prestige also increased the number of non-trauma, elective visits. What better promotional tool for any hospital, the advertising budgets of which can sometimes reach into the millions of dollars, than to have a sleek, sexy, glitzy machine sailing overhead with its logo emblazoned in high-gloss letters?

Many of the downtime duties of the nurses in Cindy's group dealt with the business side of air care. Generating feedback reports to original referral sources, be they community hospitals or surface EMS providers, was an essential ingredient. Each wanted to know the disposition of the patients they sent. In part, the reports were motivated by educational and humanitarian purposes. In part, it was basic marketing strategy.

If Hospital X has been designated as a Level I trauma center, there are a variety of community hospitals within its sphere of influence. But sitting about 160 miles to the west is competitor Hospital Z, with its own flight team and the potential to scoop up patients and revenue. If the customer isn't appropriately stroked, the next time they have a critically ill patient—or *five* critically ill patients—they may decide to give the competition a try.

As far as possible, flight teams try to keep their sources happy. It's necessary for flight nurses to establish flexible working relationships in the field, to be a diplomat when on a mission, to know when to strike up a take-charge, "everybody stand back, the flight team is here!" attitude, and to know when to sidle up to someone on-scene and say, "Hey, I'm here, could you tell me what's going on?'' The rule is to never step on toes unless the patient is being compromised by incompetence.

Numerous inducements for customer relations are used, from price undercutting through memorabilia—little helicopter pins, coffee mugs, or CPR posters—to elaborate, free in-service programs for the staff: ''Yes, thank you for calling us. Perhaps next time, if you have any questions about how to resuscitate a pediatric case, our folks would be delighted to come out. We have this free class that at any given moment one of our nurses would love to come by and share with you.''

The smaller hospitals love it.

Working with the families of those injured was a common element in Cindy's job as well. Many people need someone to translate the workings of the system for them. Contacts to assist in this often begin at the accident site, directing them to the hospital, telling them whom to contact upon arrival, even helping them find nearby lodging, if necessary.

''Here's my card. Give me a call, and I'll be able to tell you what's going on with your family member.''

There was a tremendous amount of follow-up of each case brought in by air, reams of paperwork to be processed. For instance, in the case of the truck driver, Mr. P., severe social problems existed for his wife. When Cindy stopped by the ICU after coming in from another mission, Mrs. P. was in the waiting area with her seven children, six of whom were under the age of twelve.

They were obviously indigent; they had no diapers, no shoes. They had run out of milk at home. The wife was a humble, passive person, unlikely to seek assistance. She felt totally isolated, paralyzed in her concern for her husband. They had only recently moved from the southwest and had no friends or family nearby. Cindy set about making calls to the appropriate social agencies, explaining to Mrs. P. the bureaucratic process and means of circumventing snags.

Another priority component for nurses was the maintenance of proficiency. Flight nurses practice ''extended skills,'' which need to be kept up. Performing procedures such as intubating patients, inserting femoral artery lines, or performing surgical cricothyrotomies when the upper airway is obstructed are not uncommon in fieldwork.

Another task, rarely formalized, was learning to cope with the work and living with all that is witnessed, the situations taken home to sleep with at night, and the powerlessness known to every nurse of being caught in between. . . .

The call was for a six-month-old boy. Cardiac arrest in the home. No one knew why. He had been sitting on the porch, propped up in his child seat, drinking his bottle quietly, nodding toward sleep. He snuggled into the covers as soon as he was laid down. When a family member went to check on him, he was blue, not breathing. They rushed him to the emergency department, where a pediatrician instituted resuscitation. The physician called for the flight team after several minutes of working on the child with virtually no response.

Radio transmission is often at its worst while the aircraft is setting down on the pad. None of the crew picked up that the doctor had decided to discontinue the code. When they walked through the door, he looked startled.

"Oh, God, you're here! Great, we can go ahead and transfer this kid."

Cindy and her partner quickly sized up the situation. The child had been in full arrest for an hour. It was hopeless.

"Let's be blunt, doctor," Cindy said, taking the physician aside. "This child is dead. There is no hope whatsoever of saving him. You need to call this code and put this situation to rest."

He wasn't having any of it. He wanted the child out of his service. Unself-consciously abrupt, he left to inform the family of the transfer. He had someone to dump this tragedy on.

"Cindy, we can't take this baby," Pam said. "We'll be doing CPR in flight all the way."

"I know, I know. . . ."

Cindy placed a call to their medical-control physician and related their situation, hoping for reprieve, but knowing the protocol too well.

"Well, now, Cindy, I can't really discontinue anything over the phone. You know the drill—he's the one who's with the patient. . . ."

"So, then we have to take this major catastrophe and transport it for thirty minutes? That's what you're telling me?"

"I'm sorry . . ."

She felt impotent, infuriated. She felt the fog rolling in. She wanted to turn around and throw up on the floor.

The pilot stood by, waiting, watching while Pam and Cindy began mixing solutions, hanging multiple drips, setting up the transfer gurney, passing instructions to the ER nurses, their flight suits already wringing wet.

"I have never felt so helpless," he said.

"I know." Cindy nodded.

"What can I do?"

"You can't do anything," Cindy shrugged. "But thanks."

That was the first conversation between her and her future husband.

As they exited, the hospital staff nurses continuing compressions, bagging the baby, the pediatrician returned, alone.

"Where are the parents?" Cindy demanded.

"They're back in the waiting room."

"Well, I want them to come out here."

"There's no time," he said, shooing them along. "Hurry."

"There's time!" Cindy insisted.

He tried nudging them through the doors, but she clasped its edge, lodging her hip against the gurney. "Those parents are coming out here. . . ."

"It's not even the parents. They're the grandparents. It's one of those extended family things. The mother doesn't even know yet. Nobody knows where she is. She's just a kid herself, fifteen or sixteen years old. Now, get a move on."

"I don't care *who* they are; they're family. It's important that they be with this baby before he's gone. . . . If you don't want the responsibility of pronouncing this death, so be it, but we're not going until they see this child!''

''All right, all right!'' He snapped angrily for one of the staff to bring the family. ''Now, will you get this kid on board.''

They moved the child quickly, taking over compressions from the hospital nurses, who offered apologies and wished them good luck. Maneuvering in the tiny space, trying to keep the drips going, Cindy and Pam attached the cardiac leads. The child was secured inside the cabin when the family arrived. They were a couple in their late thirties, clutching each other with that numbed, bewildered look common to the terrified.

''He's going to look different,'' Cindy said, assisting them into the cabin, directing them to the head of the bed. ''There are tubes and blood and bandages. But it's okay to touch him. That's right, you need to hold your child. . . .''

Their movements were tentative, fearful of dislodging IV lines. She urged them on, the tension welling, almost palpable in that cramped space, the rotors whipping above.

''Do you see what we're doing here? Every once in a while, I have to externally provide compressions for the heart. . . . I have to be very honest with you that I don't think your baby is going to make it. You must understand we are doing all . . .''

The woman drew in an astonished breath. She spoke slowly, as if trying to recall a dream, beginning with a phrase known to all nurses: ''*But the doctor said* you were going to save his life!''

''Well,'' Cindy stammered, stunned. ''It's just not a case of it being in our hands right now. It's much more grave a situ—''

''Yes,'' her husband nodded. ''He said you would take him to the university hospital, and they would put a pacemaker in.''

Cindy was doubly stunned, astonished at the scope of the lie, unable to respond. She tried to speak but felt sickened. There was not a hospital within hundreds of miles where such an experimental procedure would be attempted on a child of this age, even under optimal conditions.

She looked them in the eyes, shaking her head sadly. The

couple was so wracked with emotion that they fell to the floor. She helped them up, trembling herself, knowing the child would not be alive when they next saw him, imagining their tortured drive to the hospital, seeing them walk through the corridors, having to wait for the elevator to take them to the pediatric ICU, nursing their secret hopes, only to see his sweet dead body.

Cindy stood amid the fracas, choking on raw rage and revulsion, looking past the couple to the pediatrician with an expression that said, I wish I had an Uzi right now, mister, because I would torment you with it.

It took some time, but she guided them beneath the tubing and wires to where they could pick him up.

"You need to kiss your child good-bye."

The helicopter lurched with lift-off, its single engine straining upward at an angle. The couple remained statue-still, clutching each other, faces upturned, growing smaller as the helicopter rose. It was like the descriptions of after-death experiences, the soul rising away from the body.

Both she and Pam knew it was an exercise in futility, an insult to whatever life may have remained. They held their own tears in by focusing on the task at hand: bagging, compressing, checking lines—the ABCs of emergency intervention: Airway, Breathing, Circulation. The loss of a child is the ultimate loss. More than any other experience, it encourages that nagging question: What if . . . ? So they kept at it, unrelenting, working balls-to-the-walls as muscles grew to ache and the sweat ran down their flesh.

Full-scale resuscitation followed landing, without results. Cindy's supervising physician, whom she'd spoken with on the phone, approached and patted them on the back.

"Boy, that was really a heroic run."

"Doctor," Cindy ice-eyed him, motioning toward the door. "We need to go outside."

"We went under the canopy outside while I laid that man wide open. I said, 'You have no idea, as a nursing professional, what you just put me through. . . . There was no reason that had to happen!' I went on and on, all the frustration and rage and pity just gushing out of me. I saw those people and how they wept. That would be my memory. After it's all done and over and everything's gone, you're the person who's left with that, and the memory of that child.

"That affected me very deeply.

"It was a situation that just burned me out. It burned me that other forces can manipulate you. It's all a part of that political thing between doctors and nurses. So often it boils down to raw power.

"Now, when I give my lectures, I tell that story and talk about how important it is to take that thirty seconds or a minute, whatever it takes to let these family members see that person. . . . That, and, 'Don't lie to people. That's the most important thing. You are doing no one any service by lying to them.'

"That's true for nurses at the bedside, in an ER, or in the field. We're the ones who are with patients, who care about that person's emotional needs."

Cindy was in fieldwork for two years before feeling she needed a break. She could see why the military rotate flight nurses out after that amount of time. After two years, she had seen so much hurt and pain that she stopped seeing the successes. The fifty-five-hour weeks began feeling exactly like that. The difficulty of managing a personal life between shift work, sick-out coverage, and late days off the clock started gnawing her concentration.

She started looking critically at her career. There is steady pressure within the profession for nurses to attain a bachelor's degree. She had been enrolled in classes the entire time in North Carolina but missed more than she completed; when it's 7:00 P.M. and you should be punching out to go to a class at eight, but are off in East Jerusalem on an OTR, it makes for a tight fit.

"I found myself asking, 'Am I the only one seeing the bad things?' The glory had faded. It was a period of just hard, kick-ass work. You find yourself out in some Screaming Beaver in the middle of the night responding to a 1050 PI [multiple extremity amputation], turning O_2 cylinders, and your hands are so frosted that your fingers won't grip. Or you find yourself cleaning up the helicopter after a patient has puked in it, because people puke in helicopters just like they puke on the ground and in ambulances. . . . And I mean, who else is gonna do it?

"You find yourself getting angry over some minor thing like not being able to grow nails because you know they'll break off while lugging equipment around. You start thinking defensively—where will I *be* in ten years?

"Do you really want to be jumping out of helicopters when you're fifty, Cindy?

"On the other hand, you have all this autonomy and independence that you know they'd never let you exercise if you returned to hospital-staff nursing. Once you've become so autonomous, once you've been out on the road and taken charge and sharpened your assessment skills to that degree, how do you go back?"

Personal considerations ultimately decided for her. The pilot she'd been dating called one evening to tell her that the corporate office was transferring him to Montgomery, Alabama. He wanted her to come along. They decided to marry. Around the same time another nurse, Mary Jo, with whom she had started out on the team and who was eight months pregnant, finally decided it was time for maternity leave. The signs seemed right for a change.

"A week after I left, the helicopter crashed, killing everyone aboard, including Pam, my ex-roommate and flight partner. There was a fire on board. The exact circumstances were never clear, but it was an eerie, awful feeling. Had we remained on schedule, it would have been on our shift that the crash occurred. It hit the community as well as the program very hard. It broke my heart.

"I take my hat off to the people who put that program back together."

Cindy has tried to remain in some area of the aviation industry. The program she works for currently employs only paramedics in a direct flight capacity. This is a policy she has been working to change, especially in the area of inter-hospital transfers, where a paramedic's expertise is least applicable.

She has become involved in the political machinery that guides such decisions in the state. Much of her time is spent in coordinating surface and air EMS units as well as providing in-service education to hospital nursing services, instructing them on what types of patients will benefit from Medevac and what the flight crews will need to ease the transport. Her biggest stumbling blocks within hospitals are the effects the nursing shortage and recession are having on emergency departments and ICUs. Because of insufficient staff, units have been closed, transports turned away, and the entire system backed up.

From her office, she can hear the helicopters arrive and depart. She is burning to get back into the air, though she also feels valued for the information she imparts in her lectures, helping to push the bounds of her profession just a bit further.

"I recently saw a TV special about the effects of the nursing shortage on health care. What struck me was that in the first frames they showed a helicopter lifting off on a mission. You wouldn't have seen that a few years ago. But people are starting to recognize that piece of the profession now, what an integral part flight nursing has become. I was very proud."

2

"To Be Needed"

Becoming a Nurse

Dan is a burly-framed man just shy of six feet with reddish hair and beard. Before entering nursing school, he acquired a journalism degree from Ohio State. But in the wake of Watergate, the job market was horrible, overloaded with would-be Woodsteins. He wound up working as an assistant manager at K Mart.

He'd always been fascinated by TV medical documentaries; anything health- or science-related. He had a buddy in nursing school who convinced him to give it a try: it was a job guarantee forever and anywhere. For Dan, single and in his late twenties, the travel incentive was particularly appealing. His friend had followed another guy into nursing who'd done the same. They thought of themselves as a chain of guys who got one another in. Someone Dan knew from back home followed him.

Initially he entered the field because he wanted some training that could translate directly into cash. His perspective changed while he was still in school. During a clinical rotation on a medical floor, he was assigned an elderly black man who'd had a cerebrovascular accident (CVA; a stroke). Mr. D. was crumpled up from his CVA, immobile, his stony face drooping to the left side. He could look at people but was unable to say anything.

Dan's clinical instructor on that rotation was forever stressing the necessity of talking to stroke victims as if they understood what was said.

"Whether or not you know they can, you have to assume they can."

While going through his patient's history to prepare for the assignment, Dan discovered that Mr. D. was an avid baseball fan. So each clinical day, Dan brought in the newspaper box scores. He would pick Mr. D. up, bathe him, towel him off, powder, and dress him. Then he positioned him in a chair, pillows propping limbs, and read the scores to him.

On the last day of his clinical rotation on that floor, Dan said, "Mr. D., I've got to go now. I want you to know, sir, that it's been a pleasure meeting you and working with you."

This ninety-eight pound old man, who hadn't whispered a word to anyone since his stroke, drew in a deep breath and said, "Thank you."

"I was stunned. I was, like, ten feet off the ground. It made me realize that what I'd gotten into was not just a job."

Individuals are drawn to nursing along different paths. Religious and philosophical principles, family molding and societal expectations may all play a part. Sometimes it's as simple as economic necessity, one job leading to another. As with most life choices, the earlier the desire is imprinted, the less clear the motivation.

Pat wanted to be a nurse from the time she was five or six but married and started a family soon after leaving high school. The desire continued to percolate, however, and as soon as her children were in school, she enrolled in a nursing program. For the two years of her associate-degree program, she survived on minimal sleep, working a trio of eleven to seven shifts weekly as a nursing assistant while taking classes during the day and mothering in the evening.

"It was simply something I had to do. Why, I'll never know."

Doreen, today the nurse manager of a GI/endoscopy clinic in one of the largest university-based hospitals in the country, can't recall what specifically drew her to nursing. As far back as she can recall, she wanted to be one. The single association she makes is that the person she felt closest to as a youngster was her grandmother, who became very ill when Doreen was nine. She had malignant hypertension, eventually dying in renal failure.

Her grandmother was hospitalized for a long period. Doreen cared deeply for her and spent much of her free time there, fetching glasses of water, running errands, enjoying whatever little things she could do to comfort her. She came to recognize that nursing represented the nurturing part of health care, the caring aspect of care giving.

"More than anything, I would say that's where nursing's uniqueness lies. I think that's why people go into nursing, at least the ones who wind up being any good at it. I think that they, more than any other segment of the health care industry, have a tendency to see the human side of the person they're caring for and are more apt to put themselves in the patient's place. I just don't know that anybody else does that. I wanted to be a part of that caring. I guess I need to be needed."

For some, the role model of a relative or neighbor was a motivating factor. "My mother's sister was a nurse. She always seemed more self-possessed than Mom. She was single and had her own apartment. She did what she wanted. I liked that," a San Francisco clinical specialist in oncology explains. "And she always had these gruesomely funny hospital stories to tell. When we'd visit her, I used to look through her nursing books at all the photos of injuries and diseases—skin cancers, burn victims, surgical incisions. I was keenly aware of my own body and had never considered such decay possible. It used to gross my brothers out, but it was very intriguing to me."

Others were exposed to nurses through the illness of family

members or friends. When Joy, today an official of a southern state's Nurses' Association, was thirteen, a close friend was involved in an accident and ended up being paralyzed from the waist down. He was treated at a university medical center. Because he was an excellent patient for nursing students to work with, needing all the basic care—turning and positioning to avoid bedsores, assistance with hygiene and feeding, counseling for adaptation to a handicap, grief work—Joy got to know many student nurses. They were the ones who first interested her in nursing as a career.

Because nursing has traditionally been a "female profession," for many women who came of age at a certain time, it was seen as something a young woman could "fall back on," as a way of always securing a job.

"That was twenty-five years ago. There weren't many female doctors or lawyers or scientists around. At least I didn't know any. It was either be a teacher or a nurse. I was good in math and science. And I preferred to work with adults."

Even today, many define their choice in terms of an option within their grasp. A Chicago-area RN who has specialized in gerontology for three of her five years in the field states, "Nursing is a lot like being a cop or a fireman. The folks at the ANA [American Nurses' Association] might go nuts to hear this said, but nursing is a working-class profession. To me that's not a criticism. That's where I come from, and I'm proud of it."

For Ernestine, becoming a nurse was purely a matter of chance. Out of high school, she went to a large, private psychiatric facility hoping to find work as a beautician. A personnel department worker told her that the beauticians there were older than ice and had to die or retire before there would be an opening.

Sensing Ernestine's disappointment, the woman encouraged her to put in an application as a psychiatric aide. Psychiatric aides are a part of the nursing department, comparable to nursing assistants in medical hospitals—i.e., the bottom of the health care power pyramid, thus having the most direct patient contact and the least power.

A head nurse interviewed and hired her, and she started two weeks later.

After being on the unit awhile, Ernestine noticed two things: several of the psych aides had been there for twenty or thirty years, and they were both resigned and bitter about their lack of responsibility and authority in decision making. At the same time, there were student nurses who did psych rotations on the hall. Ernestine watched these students, some younger than she, pass through only to return as staff nurses making more money and having more authority.

She decided it was time to return to school.

Originally, Frank wanted to be a history teacher. His mother was a nurse, and there was a lot of illness in his family—a diabetic sister, asthmatic cousins, the early death of his father. In retrospect, he is unsure how much any of that mattered. At the time, nursing just seemed to come naturally even though men comprise only about 3 percent of the profession's ranks.

"Being a male who makes the decision to become a nurse, from jump street, you're looked at as being gay—not by immediate family, but by a few cousins and neighbors, people you meet. I grew up in a small Pennsylvania town where most people worked in a factory or as some type of laborer. It was just unheard of. I mean, if I had become a teacher, I'd have been looked at as some kind of wimp, but a nurse—Christ, there's something wrong with the boy!

"But when you put your choice of being a nurse in terms of economics and job security—I mean, I'm always going to have a job and never get laid off—then people say, 'Oh, yeah, I hadn't thought of it that way. That's a pretty good idea.'

"It also depends upon the area you choose to work in. If it's in psych or the ER, people say, 'Well, that's okay.' But if

I wanted to work in obstetrics, I'm sure people would think I was kind of strange.''

Common reasons for choosing to join this helping profession include the desire to *work with human beings rather than inanimate objects, balance sheets, or computers* and the often unexamined impulse *to do good and help others.* Typical beauty pageant slogans, right? ''Well, for me,'' Debbie says, ''they were true.''

Debbie's mother was chronically ill when she was young. Debbie spent a lot of time in hospitals, plagued by the nagging guilt children sometimes feel: ''Maybe if I knew enough, my mom wouldn't get sick.''

For some, the impulse to help may have a darker hue, recognized only with the broadening perspective of maturity. Why she chose to go into nursing is something that Vivian, twenty-six year old psychiatric nurse, has done a good bit of soul searching about. A lot of it had to do with the relationship she had with her family. As the youngest of three sisters, she was ''the Kid,'' and exempted from the burning rivalries that raged between the older two.

''I don't know what it was, but people would always tell me stuff—personal things I shouldn't have been told and really didn't want to know. Maybe it's because I have an easygoing attitude. That's genuine; I've never been judgmental. My two older sisters didn't get along, so I was always acting as a go-between. I was always 'the peacemaker,' the one who brought everybody together. I'm still that way, though my family's changed and sort of mellowed. I've become very interested in learning about 'the Dysfunctional Family,' about the one whose role it is to 'make the peace,' the one who 'takes care.' ''

When her older sisters moved out of the house, Vivi was twelve or thirteen years old. Her parents were having marital problems, and she slipped into the role of confidante, the pseudo-therapist, the adult in the relationship. Her father would take her for walks along the beach, talking about how her mother needed to feel that she was constantly loved.

She listened, not understanding most of it, but thinking, "Why is he telling *me* this?"

Then, from Mom, she heard about his infidelities, whether true or not. It was all very weird. But Vivian kept a good secret, already adept at knowing she shouldn't go running back to Mom, asking, "Dad has these feelings like you're unable to feel loved. What is *that* all about?" Looking back, she believes her mother was going through a serious depression; she would lie on the sofa daily, Vivian ministering to her needs. Dad ignored the problem, tending not to see things he preferred not seeing.

> "I'm sure my memory of things may be a little distorted, but I think the need to help people 'make it better,' to 'fix things,' and to get satisfaction from 'making things work' began for me at that time. There was a measure of control and a sense of belonging in being able to do that. Because I think I do have a knack for being approachable and trustworthy. People feel comfortable with me, safe talking to me. I'm not a very threatening person, just sort of sweet and kind."

Peggy came to nursing circuitously, by way of the convent. Her childhood dream was to become a nun. For her to be confident that entering the convent wasn't a form of escape, preacceptance qualifications included getting a job "in the world" for one year, along with completing at least one college-level course.

She was sent to the personnel department of a community hospital in the largest nearby city. Having no prior experience beyond cleaning churches and making homemade ice cream in a local parlor, she was not very hopeful. But it turned out that the head of the personnel department lived around the corner from where Peggy's family vacationed every summer. They spent the entire interview talking about the area, their shared love of the beaches, pines, and holiday celebrations. She was a shoo-in.

The job was as a nursing unit clerk in a busy emergency room. She was eighteen and outside her family circle for the first time. The nurses took her under their wing, explaining things, introducing her to attitudes and experiences never imagined, and advising her about class selections. At the end of the year, she was admitted to the convent. She was informed that she was to become a teacher.

"What I'd really like," she informed the mother superior, "is to become a nurse, because I've got some time under my belt and think I could pick it up pretty quickly."

"A commendable notion," she was assured. "But there are no openings in that area."

Peggy said, "But it's what I want to do."

Mother Superior said, "But you can't."

She tried it their way, for a year and a half, without satisfaction.

"It was this whole control thing that I didn't understand at the time. But I took up for myself and stuck with my desire to be a nurse. I had no clear idea why. I just knew the excitement in the emergency room held me. It was the quick-thinking, the fast-acting aspect of it. Also, I think it had to do with the immediate results of it. I think I function better if I'm in a crisis situation. There's immediate gratification. I don't see patients get well, but I know I've had an impact."

She went back to working in the ER full-time and enrolled in nursing school. Being next to penniless, she had to drop out two or three times, saving up for the next semester as she went. She chose a four-year university program on the advice of the ER head nurse, who said, "Do it this way, and you'll have time to figure out what you want."

It was years before she gained insight into the family dynamics that spawned her gravitation to crisis situations. Three years ago, as her mother was dying, her brother's alcoholism went full-blown. He sabotaged her and was terribly destructive to the family. Peggy came to recognize that she'd been raised in an alcoholic family, that her father was an alcoholic, that her brother is an alcoholic. She began to learn about the roles assigned and assumed in alcoholic families, patterns of co-dependence, martyrdom, and caretaking.

As often happens with family members of alcoholics, she first became involved in Al-Anon and ACOA (Adult Children of Alcoholics) in an attempt to, once again, render help to the designated drunk, only to find her own needs reflected.

"It's taken me awhile to realize it, but I believe nurses are basically co-dependent, a very co-dependent group. They forget about themselves so much. They always find a reason to do for somebody else. That was certainly my job in the family when I was young. The crisis aspect of emergency medicine plays into that perfectly. That's what the ACOA family is—a crisis family. I do crisis well. Just don't ask me to do the long-term stuff."

Anna taught high school for ten years before considering a career move. Teaching had become unreliable. The pupil population was dwindling and with it available positions. There was a money crunch, and people were being let go, even teachers with tenure. She tried other jobs—research assistant, circulation work, retail sales—but found they weren't especially fulfilling.

"There's a strong need in me to be of service, which showed up in my choice of teaching as a career and later nursing. I don't think choices are accidental."

Regardless of when or why the choice is made, the aspiring nurse faces a sometimes bewildering array of educational paths to becoming an RN. Currently there are three basic entry routes: the two-year associate degree in nursing (ADN), commonly obtained in a community college; a three-year diploma earned in a hospital-based school; and the four-year Bachelor of Science in Nursing (BSN) degree acquired in a university.

The subject of what constitutes appropriate credentials to be an RN—which program types are "better," each with its own degree of one-upmanship—is a perennially bitter controversy within the profession, at times pitting nurse against nurse. (There is even a saying summarizing these tensions: "Nursing eats its young.") The route chosen can have a reverberating impact on the nurse's career, reflected in pay scale, job openings, and even personal associations.

In 1979, Pat became a nurse practitioner. While today it is assumed that most nurse practitioners have master's degrees, at that time the criteria was that you had to be an RN with five years of critical-care experience and pass a certification exam. Over the next few years, Pat was involved in establishing a regional cardiac rehab lab, handpicking her staff, establishing guidelines, and developing programs. Each year several university nursing programs used the lab as a clinical rotation area for students. Pat enjoyed the teaching as much as the work. The students always gave the program glowing evaluations.

It was common that at the beginning of each academic year, each university would contact Pat to arrange the students' schedules. In 1987, she got such a call, and after deciding on the manageable student ratio, the head of the one university nursing office said, "Oh, by the way, we've been updating our records, and there's just one bit of information missing from your file. Where is your master's degree in nursing from?"

"Well, actually," Pat said, "I'm a certified nurse practitioner. I have an associate's degree in nursing and a bachelor's degree in communications, but I don't have a master's degree."

"Oh, well," she was told after an uncomfortable silence. "Then we won't be able to place students with you any longer."

Later that day, Pat received a call from another university nursing department wanting to know how many students she could handle.

"Listen," she interrupted. "Before we go any further, I feel I must tell you that I don't have a master's degree in nursing."

"Well, I appreciate the information, but that really doesn't matter to us. What we're interested in is that our students get the best clinical exposure they can, and you've always given them that."

Diploma programs are the remnants of a time when nurses were "trained" instead of being "educated." In that system, tasks were taught in an apprenticeship modal, the performance of rote, repetitive actions without explanation of the principle underlying the action—left hand holds this, while right hand moves that. Administrators of such programs often believed that women lacked the intelligence to grasp abstract principles, obviating the need to give such instruction. Hospital-diploma schools existed to train workers to staff hospital wards, period, and to do so as cheaply as possible.

In the beginning of this century, a nursing-reform movement began placing emphasis on nurses being broadly educated and attaining a baccalaureate degree in the belief that this was necessary to enable nursing to hold a distinct standing as a profession, "to professionalize the profession." As the century progressed, with the erosion of numerous social institutions and individuals becoming known less for who they were or where they came from and more for what they did, the initials after someone's name acquired added currency as a marker of social expectation and trust.

Associate-degree programs arose in the early 1950s. The Cadet Nurse Corps, created to meet nursing needs during World War II, confirmed that students could attain clinical proficiency in less than three years. This coincided with the rise of community colleges across the country, often drawing older students into practice. At the inception of AD programs, these nurses were conceived to be more technician-like, acting under the direction of BSN grads. In reality, though, this distinction was never applied in the field.

Whatever type of program a student attends, upon completion of all classes and clinical rotations she or he is considered a graduate nurse, a GN. She/he is able to practice in this legally limited capacity until sitting for a nationally standardized examination, NCLEX, administered by each state's Board of Nursing, commonly referred to as state boards. (Failure to pass the exam on the first try necessitates relinquishing GN status, though the aspirant nurse may sit for the exam whenever it is offered until she or he passes.) The NCLEX is a two-day, eight-hour test ranging over all aspects of nursing practice. Passing it grants the title registered nurse, RN. Thus, all RNs enter the workplace with equal marketability.

The animosities that spring from these three types of degrees coexisting side by side tend to run in stereotypic fashion: diploma nurses—with the most in-depth clinical background but the least academic credit—graduate with superior technical skills, allowing them to fit more easily into the workplace. They tend to sneer at BSN grads, whom they view as being strong in the snob-factor of leadership skills but unable to hold their own when it comes to performance.

Barbara, a diploma grad, worked in a university hospital for several years where she commonly encountered BSN grads groomed to manage a unit. Unfortunately, they were working as staff nurses and couldn't do any of those things they felt competent to manage, having been taught that such tasks were beneath them.

"I'd be making up the assignment sheet at the beginning of a shift—and it was common practice for each nurse to be expected to care for eight or more patients—and these BSNers would actually tell me, 'Oh, I can only do two patients. I was taught to care for the patient's psychological needs and render a lot of emotional support, so I don't have time to do all those "tasky" things, like back rubs and bedpans.'

"Well, excuse me, but when somebody needs a bedpan, they don't want to talk about how they *feel* about needing the

bedpan; they just want the bedpan. And I'm s
be verified through research. I've had occasion whe
haste, I asked a BSN grad to give a patient a bedpan and b
told, 'Oh, I'm not here to do that.'

"Personally, I have never, ever considered *any* task as being beneath me in rendering care for a patient. If I had time
or could do it, I would do it. Otherwise, I'd ask somebody to
help.''

BSN grads tend to disparage diploma and ADN grads as
drones unable to conceptualize the holistic psychosocial needs
of patients. Gail, a master's-prepared nursing instructor, thinks
that diploma nurses should be dumped entirely, believing they
are a negative weight against the struggles of the profession to
gain greater respect. While working in Tennessee in the late
1980s, she was aghast to meet recent diploma grads who'd been
trained to stand up whenever a doctor walked into the room.
She believes ADN graduates should be relegated to the technician status for which they were created. Joyce, a generic BSN
graduate in 1970, never gave a thought to going to diploma
school. For her, it made no sense to go to school for three years
and receive only a certificate that, according to society's standards, meant little when she could go to college for another year
and earn a degree. She saw diploma students as being rewarded
not to think, but to fit into a mold.

"That's not an indictment; it's a reflection of where women
were at that time, where the practice of medicine and health
care was at that time.''

It has been said that diploma students are taught to think the
doctor is God, while BSN students are taught to think that they
are God.

Perhaps because the average ADN student is thirty years old,
those interviewed tended to approach the issue from a pragmatic
point of view, having matriculated into a two-year program be-

to entering the work force, thus
than paying to learn. At a cost of
lars and as much as two more years
BSN seemed questionable at best. In
azine reported that BSN grads who work
hourly difference of eighty cents more than
AD nty cents less than diploma nurses. Dan ech-
oes a co pinion:

> "Nurses are always getting into all this diploma versus ADN
> versus BSN crap. Clinically, if you're comparing an ADN to
> a BSN, they're essentially the same. If you're talking about
> how either prepares you for what goes on in the actual hospital
> setting, they're both jokes. The real learning goes on your
> first couple of years in practice, after you've got an RN. You
> may get a taste of it when you do clinicals, but in that first
> year you're not worth a damn. You're not worth your salt. It's
> only after some hard-core experience that you grow."

Nursing education tends to be broken into two facets—the didactic, philosophical realm and hands-on patient contact in clinical rotations. Philosophies of nursing differ between schools,
but there are some common elements. Curricula usually include
courses in anatomy and physiology, chemistry (organic and in-
organic), biology, biochemistry, growth and development, nutrition, math, statistics, psychology, sociology, nursing ethics,
and professional issues. More and more there are also courses
in management techniques and data processing. As the slogan
of a national nursing image-enhancing campaign launched in
early 1990 states: "If caring was all it took, anyone could be a
nurse."

Of course, the essential goal of nursing school is being socialized as a nurse, from mastering multiple treatment tasks to
acquiring a philosophy of nursing. Homeostasis, the self-
regulatory balance within a person (or any system) that allows
it to function optimally, is a key concept in the philosophical

base of nursing. Students are encouraged to view their work as both a science and an art; bringing science to bear on correcting a problem while employing the artfulness of human contact, the therapeutic use of the self, to maintain or replenish the homeostatic balance of each individual patient. A high premium is placed upon helping people maintain wellness through healthier life-style choices and preventive practices.

"Care, not cure" is a phrase often applied to nursing. It is the province of medicine to diagnose and treat illness. It is the province of nursing to deal with the person who has that illness. Nursing programs stress the concept of holistic care of individuals, ideally viewing each patient within the context of his or her physical, psychosocial, and spiritual needs. Students are sensitized to patient dependency and vulnerability, persons stripped of their individuality and dignity when clothing is exchanged for a hospital gown. They are taught to identify and assist patients with their *responses* to illness—their fear and confusion, anxiety and frustration, their hope, helplessness, and despair. They likewise acquire the nomenclature of misery-mitigating, pain-cheapening words—discomfort, morbidity, mortality—that buffer the shocks of witnessed reality.

There is a saying: "The purpose of medicine is to diagnose and treat disease. The purpose of nursing is to do everything else." To accomplish nursing treatment goals, the "nursing process," a four-step variation on the "scientific method," is employed: assessment (collecting data about patient problems and needs); analysis and planning interventions; implementing plans; and evaluating the outcome. This is formulated into a nursing care plan (NCP) consisting of four parts. First, a nursing diagnosis—something like "potential for injury, related to patient confusion manifested by patient's belief that he is at home and attempting to climb over side rails." Next, the expected outcome, which is supposed to be realistic with measurable goals—i.e., "Patient will remain free from injury while hospitalized or until confusion resolves." Third, nursing interventions to accomplish the goal—use of Posey to keep patient in bed, frequent conversation to help reorient patient, etc. Finally, an evaluation after a few days to assess the efficacy of plans.

Nursing care plans form the basis of nursing documentation in hospitals. It is a format recognized and reinforced by the Joint Commission on the Accreditation of Healthcare Organizations (JCAHO) when evaluating institutions and is increasingly tied to insurance reimbursement for services. (Accreditation is a voluntary program, hospitals paying to be surveyed by the Joint Commission to make sure that standards of care are adhered to at an acceptable level. However, without accreditation most hospitals would not receive third-party payments or meet licensure requirements. The JCAHO board is composed of twenty-four members, the vast majority from medical organizations. For years, they have denied the American Nurses' Association's petitions for board representation.)

Undergraduate nursing students are trained to be generalists, able to adapt to various clinical situations. Competence in diverse areas is expected: interpretation of lab values, physical and psychological patient assessment, evaluating medical orders, documenting what is done in a legally accountable manner, administering medications (adult and pediatric doses), and knowing the therapeutic ranges for each, running and reading EKGs, giving injections, starting IVs, drawing blood, performing sterile dressing-change techniques, and avoiding the spread of infection through habitually washing one's hands raw.

Fundamentals of nursing are relayed both in lecture form and in hands-on practice, often in simulation laboratories (sim labs) before being admitted into clinical rotations. The nondidactic, clinical component of nursing education takes place in a variety of health care facilities—hospitals, nursing homes, clinics, and home health agencies. When Joy was instructing psych, she used to take her students on a tour of the local prison so they could compare it with the state psychiatric hospital where they did their rotation. Students were usually appalled that the prison was so much nicer. Aside from having to stand outside their cell doors to be counted three times each day, prisoners could do pretty much as they pleased. Here there were murderers, rapists, arsonists, and armed robbers who had TV sets, a weight room, a running track, and other exercise facilities, a great library, fairly good food, and private cells. The psych patients, however, who'd done nothing to society other than be plagued by a painful illness, had conditions that were so overcrowded, they slept on cots in the halls and were lucky to have one TV per unit.

Clinical rotations are where nursing students get the first taste of what their careers may offer, learning what can't be conveyed in a textbook. "Clinical," as used by students, is both noun and verb; a place they go for limited exposure to learning opportunities in a variety of specialities—public health, pediatrics, medical-surgical nursing, psychiatry, labor and delivery, etc.— and something they do. Students refer to clinical rotations in terms reminiscent of "doing time" in prison: "I did my peds." "I'm doing nursery." It is where the concrete focus of nursing, helping people, is glimpsed, where theory becomes action, the words become flesh.

More than anything, Mary Beth recalls being surprised by the sights and odors of illness, the sickly decay of disease and disuse. She remembers, as if it was yesterday, helping "groom" her first colostomy. The first whiff of putrefaction knocked her off center. The sight of feces being wiped from the pink, raw bowel opening on the woman's abdomen had her stomach churning, her eyes watering. She tried to maintain composure in that dry-heave moment, hoping she wouldn't puke in front of the patient, praying her instructor would not witness her gags. She was nauseous every morning while walking to her clinical rotations just thinking about what awaited her.

Clinical is a commonly intimidating experience. For many, it is largely unpleasant and stressful, often compared to military boot camp in its rigidity. There is little room for error. In Gail's BSN program, students didn't even have sim labs to practice skills before doing them on people. They were required to read about a procedure the night before, explain it to the instructor, and go into the patient's room and perform.

"It was very scary. And truly ridiculous. I couldn't even learn to knit that way."

Students are vulnerable to the whims of clinical instructors who possess the power to snuff out their careers. Frank's program was in a religious-based school with very strict rules. Clinical pre-conference was called each morning at six-thirty, when an inspection was held to make sure uniforms were properly crisp and creased, shoes spotless, and that pens and treatment paraphernalia were secured in the appropriate pocket. For Anna, after a decade of teaching high school history, it was very distressing to know that appearance weighed as heavily as performance in whether or not she would even continue in the program long enough to be passed on to the next ordeal.

Clinical experiences often challenge whatever perceptions students bring with them. Michele arrived with notions common to the general public: that hospitals are orderly institutions run for the public good. That doctors, in particular, are professional, wise, and compassionate. Then she was pulled into an operating room on her first clinical rotation to assist with administering an epidural, a type of regional anesthesia that numbs the lower part of the body but allows the patient to remain conscious. An extra pair of hands was needed to help steady a woman being readied for a C-section. Once the anesthetic was administered, Michele helped reposition the patient and stood around waiting for it to take effect.

It was a typical OR scene, endless stainless-steel surfaces, everyone in gowns and masks, hair nets and latex gloves, the only body part exposed being everyone's eyes. The atmosphere was far more casual than what she'd seen on TV, everybody joking and generally ignoring the patient, waiting for the Betadine to dry at the incision site. It was a teaching situation, and the supervising surgeon in particular was working the room like a master of ceremonies. His OR cap was very loose, his longish hair swaying to and fro above the supposedly sterile zone. His mask, held up by one hand, was untied behind his head, and he kept dropping it down when he laughed. The patient's presence seemed entirely incidental to the rollicking good time being had by all.

The team was about to start cutting, the scalpel poised over this woman's abdomen, when she adjusted her position slightly. Everyone caught their breath, all eyes becoming the size of snowballs. Obviously, the anesthetic hadn't taken effect. The only one breathing calmly was the patient, who had no idea she'd almost been carved on while awake.

"Ah, Mrs. J.," the anesthesiologist very casually said. "Would you just raise your left leg a bit."

"Sure," she said. Up it went to a forty-five degree angle.

The guy who was to do the cut was trembling. The procedure was not only his first C-section but his first surgical incision. His supervisor stepped in, whispering, coaching him about keeping cool, while the anesthesiologist, again very matter-of-factly, explained to Mrs. J. that at this point he thought it best that they switch to general anesthesia.

"Whatever you think is best, Doctor," she said cheerily.

She went right out, and the anesthesiologist said, "Ladies and gentlemen, the clock is running. Get to work."

Martha, a BSN student, was involved with a small group of people who held each other accountable for spiritual discipline. She liked watching and talking to people and found that others sought her out to discuss their concerns. She felt she was a good listener and enjoyed helping them think through problems. She wanted to work in a counseling role and considered becoming a clinical psychologist, which could take about eight years. She wasn't sure she could last that long in school. Discovering that nurses could play the counseling role and do so much sooner, she entered nursing school specifically to work in the field of psychiatric nursing. She hoped to do outpatient therapy, believing that is where long-term change would occur.

Having been exposed to the severity of mental illnesses in her psych rotation, she is reconsidering that responsibility. She has seen how dependent patients become upon therapists, how they unrealistically idolize them.

"I've seen them do it with inpatient nursing staff, too, but there it can be deflected easier. Being the only person for them as a therapist feels heavier. There's this patient I have in my psych rotation, who's a forty-year-old woman with kids of her own, who wants to be little. She'll say that—'I wanna be little. I don't want to be big.' She feels she's about five years old.

"All this woman talks about is her ex-therapist, who means everything to her. She wants her to be her mother and take care of her forever.

"I've heard different stories about her therapist. The therapist is a woman who quit because she had a baby and needs to take care of her daughter. You can imagine how that went over with the patient. She hates the baby, talks about murdering her. The therapist used to read her bedtime stories and tuck her in. I thought it sounded pretty crazy, but the staff people say it is true.

"I'm not real sure I'd want someone being that dependent on me."

With broadening clinical exposure, students sometimes begin to question just what they've gotten themselves into. At Judyth's school in Virginia, students were given the opportunity to work for money in clinical areas for the hospital after completing each segment of the sophomore curriculum. Judyth took advantage of that after finishing her OR rotation, but only briefly. On one of her first shifts on the burn unit, everyone called in sick. It wound up being just her, a resident, and a nurse's aide for the entire shift. Burns bypassed the emergency room, and they got two admissions. She fought her inclination to flee and helped as best she could.

Nobody died as a result, but the experience scared her terribly. That was her last student employment until after graduation. She had classmates who had similar experiences who rose above them, but she concluded she didn't need that degree of stress just yet.

Before going to nursing school, Penny earned a BA in American Studies, a safe choice for someone right out of high school with a strong liberal arts background. The program offered maximum freedom: students designed their own program centered around American culture. She knew she could shine at it. Give her something where she could read a book and write a paper making comparisons with something else, and she was home free.

About halfway through college, after taking multiple social science courses, she got the idea of doing something involving the public. She knew she didn't want to sit in an office all day, to be stuck in the whole office-dress routine. She considered social work, physical therapy, and art therapy before looking into nursing. It struck her that there was so much more flexibility to mold something of one's own in nursing. There were aspects of all these professions in nursing, and the specificity of tracking was far less rigid.

To convince herself that she wasn't hiding out in academia, she decided to work for a year after graduation, taking positions as a clerical worker in an office and as a waitress. She would later joke that if you combined those jobs, you got a pretty good definition of a nurse.

After considering the different degree options, she chose a diploma school for its experiential allure, wanting to get into clinical situations as soon as possible, even if that meant doing only bed baths and taking vital signs. She wanted to taste the reality of it, to be there, assuming that if she didn't like it, she would bail out after the first year.

"One thing that drew me into nursing, I have to admit it, is that there's a curiosity aspect to my personality. In nursing school, I liked to watch codes and assist with some of the invasive procedures. I know that's really awful-sounding, but where else can you see that and have an excuse to be there? I've never seen anything like that before. I never even took shop or Home-Ec in school. I never took anything that was hands-on and physical."

However, she couldn't simply observe and remain detached from the unpleasantness; some of it pierced and clawed and latched on. Penny was still in school when her first patient died, a week after she'd cared for her. She was an elderly black woman, diabetic, hypertensive, and very depressed. They had talked a lot. She told Penny that the Lord was going to come and take her, said death would be a blessing. She was a real human being with hopes, dislikes, dreams, friends, and people who'd loved her in the past.

Three students were called in to observe when the code was called, the euphemistic "Dr. Blue." They worked on her for half an hour using chest compressions, cardiac injections, and paddle shocks that made her body bounce on the table. She died anyway.

"It sickened me to think that watching this woman die was part of my education, a check off on a Clinical Goals sheet, somebody's child, somebody's mother. I really liked her. I felt so dirty. Still, you know you have to do it so you don't fall apart when you're out there and have to be in charge. In the classroom, they talk about 'death with dignity,' then call in a couple students to watch the show. . . ."

For most students, having a patient die in front of them is a big step. For Michele it was numbing, like being in a fog afterward. The patient was a Caucasian male in his sixties who smoked several packs of cigarettes daily. He had been one of her patients earlier in the year, on the oncology floor. His lung cancer had metastasized to his liver and lymphs. From there it colonized his body.

Had she not known he was the same person, Michele wouldn't have recognized him. He'd gone downhill quickly and had been in a coma for over a week, barely clinging to a flimsy thread of life. All he could do was moan from time to time, thrash his limbs, and jerk his head back and forth. Decerebrate motion: the pointless motor spasms families always hope indicate consciousness.

Since she had last seen him, he'd turned a bright, jaundiced orange and had massive ascites, a condition in which excess fluid infiltrates the cavity containing the abdominal organs. He looked as if someone had stuck a barrel beneath the skin of his chest and belly, or blown him up like a Macy's Thanksgiving float.

It was assumed at the beginning of the shift that he would not last the day. Most of his care consisted of comfort measures and some hygiene. His floor nurse was intently concerned that all possible comfort measures were being used. She argued with his doctor all morning, on the phone and in person, lobbying to administer more analgesia.

The doctor was concerned about overmedicating, suppressing the patient's respiratory system, pushing him over the edge. As if it mattered at that point.

Just after lunch, he started to bottom out, gurgling, sputtering up bile and bleeding from his nose. Michele was in the room checking one of the numerous tubes and catheters coming out of him when it started. His whole body began quaking. She was trying to wipe him up, hearing his rasping airway work, but wondering if she needed to start suctioning. She knew the man was a DNR (Do Not Resuscitate), but wanted to call in the cavalry. She was feeling totally ineffectual, and thankful for the curtains that hid her from view, when she noticed his wife sitting motionless in the corner shadows, wringing a handkerchief, staring flatly at them.

"I know he looks bad, but he's been through this before," his wife said with such serenity that Michele felt a shiver pass through her; so *this* is what they call denial. "Once before they told me that he wouldn't make it, and he just snapped out of it."

Michele stood still, planted, staring at her with a towel full of blood in her hand from this man, feeling his death quakes and shivers as he started spewing out a throatful of black, viscous slop it would take a chemist to identify, and wanting to say, Lady, listen, he's not gonna be snapping out of this one. Instead, as calmly as she could—as much to relieve her own feelings of witnessed inadequacy as to get any help for him— she asked, "Would you mind stepping outside and asking his floor nurse to come back in?"

The floor nurse pulled the curtain entirely around the bed. She and Michele cleaned him up, the nurse speaking soothingly to him, telling him her prayers were with him, informing him his family had been called and was coming, assuring him that it was all right to let go. Then she brought his wife in and encouraged her to say whatever she felt hadn't yet been said, telling her the end was very near. The wife sat on the bed, holding his hand while she spoke, and whispered fragments of sentences between painful pauses. "I'm here, honey. It's okay, I'm right here beside you." Other family members arrived and were led in. Then he died.

After a few minutes of tears and hugs, they all stepped outside. The physician came and spoke to the family in the hall while Michele assisted with preparing the body for the morgue, disconnecting IV lines and catheters, washing and wrapping him into a bundle.

All the while his floor nurse talked about her concern that they had not done enough to alleviate his suffering. She spoke in that same soothing, respectful tone, thankful at least that the family had arrived to make it a good death, not leaving him alone among strangers at the end. She addressed Michele like an equal, thanking her for helping and assuring her that she could skip this part of it if she wished. But Michele chose to stay and help. It was the final hour of her last clinical day, senior year, spring semester. She felt a part of it now.

"Afterward everything was so real; senses heightened. It's like in death the world opens up, and you realize how precious every piece of it is, how much we take for granted. The particular becomes very real. You're very much aware of where you are—the fabric of your uniform, the lurch of the elevator, the sidewalk bustle of all that is alive around you, the brightness of the sun. It was a gorgeous day, which only made it more surreal.

"You wonder how you'll talk to anybody at home about this. It's not the kind of thing your eighteen- and nineteen-year-old friends who are studying liberal arts will relate to.

"Then, slowly, perspective returns."

Sometimes a student's clinical experience may be what nudges her toward choosing an area of specialization. Gail feels she probably ended up working in psych because she hated doing physical things like irrigating colostomies and inserting catheters. Also, because she came from a very modest home, the sight of naked people was very upsetting to her at the age of nineteen. Sticking things in people, like suctioning an airway or starting IVs, wasn't something she enjoyed either. She was afraid of it, and nobody ever helped her feel otherwise.

She decided to go into psych, however, *despite* her rotation. Due to intructor/staff infighting, the Bachelor of Science nursing school Gail attended had been barred from bringing students into the local mental hospital. Therefore, the school did its psych rotations on an outpatient basis. Students were sent into the community to do home visits with little preparation—students, alone, doing psych home visits. Gail had two patients. One wound up being very positive, a phobic woman whom she was able to follow for two semesters, getting to know her for a full academic year. Gail considered it a gift the school gave her.

The other patient, though, was a woman who lived with her daughter, both intensely impaired individuals. At her first home visit—which she had a hell of a hard time even getting to, having to take umpteen buses and subways across Boston—they were fighting with each other. The house was a shambles, smelling of decaying food and feces. Clothing and cigarette butts were strewn about. A terrier barked incessantly from the kitchen, clawing the door.

Gail talked to them briefly. She doesn't recall what it was about, something she doubtlessly thought insightful at the time, trying to intervene therapeutically, diffuse the situation. Then the daughter, never once having ceased movement, whipped out a carving knife, ripped the phone out of the wall—Gail standing there aghast, mumbling, "But, but, you can't *do* that!"—and started threatening her mother.

She never pointed the knife at Gail—this was a private pas de deux—but Gail was scared to death. The daughter kept yelling at her mother, "I'm gonna kill you, you bitch! This time I'm gonna kill you!"

And her mother, who had a broken leg in a cast, kept screaming back, "So, kill me then, kill me, you worthless kid!"

That's how Gail left them.

She ran to the subway and called her instructor, who couldn't be found. Instructors were always supposed to be available when students were out on assignment. So she called another instructor and asked if she should call the police.

He said, no, he'd call the psychiatrist, took her phone booth number, and asked her to wait. After endless minutes, he called back and told her not to worry, that this was just how this family was. They did this routinely.

Eventually, it was decided that students should not return there.

Clinical is where students become most aware that very soon they will no longer be students, but real *nurses* with the responsibility to handle such situations head-on.

3

"The Rubber Clause"

Beginning as a Nurse

"There's this nursing school mentality when you first get into practice that you'll have eight hours with two patients on a regular med-surg floor whom you can share meaningful time with, talking to and teaching them about their illness and medications, compassionately assisting them through this time of trial. Then, all of a sudden, you're out there in the real world, and you have eight or ten patients whom you're lucky to have the time to get procedures done for.

"That talk and teach stuff just says good-bye."

If nursing school is comparable to boot camp, the floor nurse is the foot soldier on the front line, the grunt walking the perimeter. Hospital floor nurses are what most people think of when they think of nurses. They are the people commonly portrayed on TV and in films, usually in the background, part of the atmosphere, associated with starched white uniforms and caps. As primary hands-on care givers, staff-level nursing is where the majority of nurses spend their careers. In 1988, two-thirds of all RNs employed in the U.S. worked in hospitals, 66.9 percent in staff-level positions.

A hospital *floor* generally refers to a medical-surgical inpatient area with private or semiprivate patient rooms. A *unit* refers to speciality areas such as intensive care, coronary care, etc. In psychiatric facilities, these terms tend to be used interchangeably along with the more archaic designations of ward or hall.

Traditionally, inpatient hospital medical-surgical floors are where the majority of nurses begin their careers. Even nurses who intend to spend their careers in psychiatric nursing are encouraged to first work a year on a general med-surg floor. It is where dues are paid and competence gained.

First jobs are where the graduate nurse (GN) encounters *reality shock*, the collision between nursing school ideals (focused on offering holistic care for the psychosocial-physio-spiritual needs of each patient) and institutional expectations (focused on the orderly completion of specific tasks, around-the-clock staffing priorities, interpersonal and interdepartmental turf boundaries, philosophical and funding disputes). Reality shock is a topic much discussed in nursing school, the subject of lectures, anecdotes, and articles. Students are warned about the transitional problems they'll encounter when they first start to practice. Still, most are not prepared for it, the real thing being a frequent rude awakening.

Mary Beth was disillusioned before her state board results arrived. Graduating with a BSN, she went to work as a GN in a labor and delivery unit. She was eager, idealistic: "Okay, world, here I am, ready to help people." She had spent four years of her life gaining specialized knowledge enabling her to assist in the delivery of babies into the world, safeguarding mother and child, able to handle unforeseen emergencies with speed and assurance.

Soon she was on the night shift, learning the ramifications of every job because she was the only one there to do them, discovering she was even expected to scrub the floor after deliveries.

> "It knocked me out, having to fold linen and mop the floor. I felt like a friggin' chambermaid."

For Joyce, nothing typified the clash between a diploma-prepared head nurse and a baccalaureate new grad than her first position, where she was chastized for not cleaning the window-sills. It had never entered her mind that cleaning windowsills would be part of her responsibilities. Yet that was so clearly a part of the head nurse's perception of nursing practice that they were like people from two different cultures talking to each other.

Numerous negotiations are necessary when a person comes into any new position. Carving out a professional identity that is distinct from other disciplines is one of the first phases of a new nurse's career. Regardless of the philosophical foundation laid in school, first jobs are where new nurses start to form a sense of what it means to be a nurse, often beginning with confronting what one doesn't know. Karen, a BSN grad, recalls her discomfort at being told to shave a patient and having to ask for instruction, never once having done the procedure in school. Debbie graduated from nursing school in 1969, the third class of an ADN program. At the time there was still confusion about the qualifications of an ADN grad. The market wasn't quite sure what to do with one. She knew herself that she didn't feel secure enough to practice safely. The first thing she did was to obtain malpractice insurance. Thankfully, she has never had to use it.

Debbie requested a position in med-surg but was told there were no openings. She was assured that as soon as one became available, she could move there, a story most staff nurses have heard at least once in their careers. Of course, it never happened.

She was placed in labor and delivery, a very intimidating place to start. Her exposure to clinical situations in nursing school had been slim. She had never done an OR rotation, never catheterized anyone, had given only a few IM injections—three or four, tops. Wanting to be forthright about her paucity of skills, she approached the head nurse.

"I'm gonna need some supervision with a few procedures, like catheterization," she said, knowing that on labor and delivery, urinary caths were as common as handshakes at a convention.

The head nurse was impassive.

"You can write RN behind your name the same as anyone else here, can't you?"

"What do you mean?" Debbie asked.

"You're a nurse," she responded, and walked away.

Debbie stood there, stung, thinking, Well, what the hell are you gonna do *now*, Deb? She doesn't know what to do with you, and you don't know what to do with her.

She was assigned to the OR suite where cesarean sections were performed. She was permitted to observe the scrub nurse once before being expected to scrub. As she stood outside the OR suite, scrubbing at the basin, her eyes filled with tears around her mask. She was thinking, Oh, God, what'm I doing here? when a kindly older OB man sidled up to scrub.

"What's the matter, hon?"

"I've never scrubbed on a C-section," she sniffled.

"Ah, don't worry about it," he assured her, lathering his arms to his elbows. "Your OR experience will stand you in good stead."

"But, you don't understand," Debbie choked. "I've never *had* any OR experience."

She could read the skepticism in his silence. At that time, it was unheard of for a nurse not to have had months of OR time while in school.

Finally, he asked, "Do you know a Kelly from a thumb forceps?"

"Yeah . . . a thumb's got a tooth in it, right?"

"You know a scalpel from a hemastat?"

"Yeah."

"Good . . . Don't worry, now, we'll take it slow. I'll tell you how to time what you need, and you just get it ready for me."

Throughout the operation, he was like molasses: *"In five . . . minutes, Debbie, I'm . . . gonna . . . need . . . a . . . clamp. . . ."* But he talked her through it without faltering.

She came to the point of really liking to scrub, appreciating the exactness of it, taking pride in her proficiency. As a head

nurse on a psych unit years later, when things would get stressful
and very vague, she would dream she was back scrubbing up
and slapping instruments—simple, precise, and predictable.

There were five other staff nurses she worked with, graduates
of three-year diploma programs, who basically said, "Debbie,
if you want to learn, shut up and watch, and we'll teach you."
They did. And did a very good job of it. The group worked
together for six months before the first one left. Today, none
of them works in labor and delivery, but they continue to
meet twice a year for dinner, including one year when Debbie
lived in California, one was in Tulsa, and another in western
Pennsylvania.

> "Baptism by fire; it bonds you. It was my first understand-
> ing of what collegiality could be. But, at the time, the mis-
> erable part was knowing that I was supposed to be taking care
> of patients and unsure how, knowing that if I screwed up, we
> could wind up with a kid who had too much oxygen, ending
> up blind. . . . Or giving penicillin and damaging an infant's
> leg permanently . . . Or not recognizing a bleed when I saw
> one, like when the fundus was getting soft . . .
> "All of that was really scary."

It is unlikely that anybody in any profession is truly prepared
for the real thing, but getting a foothold can be particularly
difficult for a new nurse. Explanations of nursing's unique characteristics center on being the caring aspect of care giving, placing oneself in the patient's place, seeing the human side of the
person being cared for.

Doctors appear on floors for brief visits, observe, probe, write
orders, and depart. Nurses are the people who are *there*, delivering that care. They are the ones with the most direct contact
with patients, introducing them to a foreign, even hostile environment—what this machine does, what that tube is for, what
can be anticipated during a treatment—and hopefully decreasing
fears and feelings of being dehumanized. The physician may be

the best orchestrator of care in the world, but if there isn't someone to perform the work, then what's the point? Nurses see
themselves as bringing the human touch to the recovery process.

Caring, comfort, support, and *reassurance*—the traditional
hallmarks of nursing practice—are difficult concepts to quantify.
It makes being a nurse a vague proposition. Certain areas, usually centering around legal aspects of practice such as medication administration and responsibility for patient safety, are very
clear. However, within a hospital hierarchy, with its layers of
power and accountability, nursing is the one group that overlaps
into every other discipline, even when it comes to performance
of tasks.

Every job has its hidden expectations and off-line account-
abilities, but many nurses believe it is this very vagueness that is
the unique feature of nursing. It could be formalized as Nursing's First Law of Overlap: Hospital staff nurses pick up the
slack, filling whatever speciality deficiencies or discrepancies
there are in the service of others. If there isn't anybody to transfer a patient, the nurse does it. Dietary workers exist to serve
trays and clear them away, but if they have not done so—or if
the patient falls through the cracks during admission or when
off the floor for a test—the nurse fills that gap. If someone needs
chest percussion or suctioning, but respiratory can't make it for
another hour and a half while the patient is turning blue, then
the nurse becomes the respiratory therapist, performing those
functions.

Anna, today a nurse practitioner, remembers her tenure as a
staff nurse well.

"PT [physical therapy] is closed on Sundays. You're with
a patient who is stiffening up, so you become PT and perform
the range of motion. . . . If you're short a nursing assistant,
then you give the bath. . . . If the family needs information
and there's no social worker around, it falls to you. . . . When
a patient has died or is dying, it's not unusual that you'll sub
for the pastoral counselor. . . . And there is no shortage of

questions from patients that their doctor should have addressed with them.

"My favorite is housekeeping. If they are there or not and a patient soils on the floor, housekeeping will not mop until the nurse has 'prepared the surface,' by which they mean she's cleaned up the stool or what have you, so they can run their little machine.

"Whatever can't, or won't, be done by somebody else, that's what nursing does. Everybody else has the right to say, 'Not my job . . .' 'I don't do trays. . . . ' 'I'm running around with my oximiter [used to measure the amount of oxygen in blood] here. How can you even *ask* me . . . ?'

"I don't know anything that a nurse can refuse to do. Many times it's even written into the contract: 'The nurse will do . . .' and they'll list forty-seven functions, the last one being, 'And other duties as directed.' There's always some rubber clause. I think that's unique to nursing. Everybody else has it pretty much nailed down."

This is a perception that has been validated by impartial investigators. A 1988 study by the Hay Group, a management consulting firm, estimated that only 26 percent of an RN's time is spent in performing "professional nursing functions." The federal panel investigating the nursing shortage reported that, "Because of the RN's versatility . . . hospitals find them to be a bargain. When needed, RNs can substitute for staff with other speciality skills as well as for less skilled staff."

Historically, physicians have been the primary power base in any hospital. While this standing has been on the wane in many places, the practice of medicine remains synonymous with health care. Because medicine and nursing are bound by function, if not always philosophy, a state akin to an uneasy truce often exists between them. Some doctor-nurse combinations are wonderful, some are workable, and some are woeful. How each individual comes to grips with this can go a long way toward dictating the ease or difficulty in getting through each shift.

Lena, an RN since 1985, works in a large university medical center in a midsize southern city. On her floor, interns are the primary doctors. They're fresh out of medical school and have the main responsibility for the patients. Intern rotations last a year. Initially, they're excited and fresh. Even if they don't know what they're doing, their intentions are good. They depend a great deal on the nurses during their first few months, which Lena appreciates. After six months, though, they can become pretty bigheaded. She has seen them go from valuing nursing input to totally ignoring any suggestions or observations.

Every nurse has at least one doctor horror story. Some see the conflict between doctors and nurses as a power relationship. Because a doctor has the greater share of power, his ability to abuse power is more pronounced, the mistakes he makes more profound. Others describe the tension in terms of sexism, each group reflecting societal roles and expectations, the "male profession" of medicine assuming carte blanche over the "female profession" of nursing.

Cathy once needed to write a note on a chart, one of a dozen or so an attending physician had taken to do rounds. Instead of waiting around an hour or so until rounds were over, she retrieved the one she needed and proceeded with her work. The physician found her and asked if she'd taken it. When she handed it to him, he slapped her on the hand, told her she was a bad girl, and said if she did it again he'd have to spank her. She was flabbergasted and insulted. She complained to her head nurse, the shift supervisor, and eventually her assistant director of nursing. There were several witnesses, none disputing her description of events. It supposedly bounced around in several interdepartmental hearing committees, but nothing ever came of it, not even an apology.

Pat, today a nurse practitioner, believes the doctor-nurse game is an improving situation, directly as the result of assertiveness training. Nurses are less likely to be intimidated by physicians simply because of title or gender, and expect to be taken seriously as people and professionals. A few years ago, she wrote a paper called "Nursing's Struggle: A Woman's Problem." It was inspired by an incident she endured with a clinic physician at her hospital who was well known for his explosive temper, particularly toward nurses. He'd curse out any nurse, regardless of who was present.

Pat was working on a cardiac floor when she received a call from his secretary informing her that this doctor wanted to see her downstairs in his clinic, "STAT." She went down to the clinic, unable to guess what he might want. A man lay on a stretcher in the hall, quite conscious. The doctor stood beside him, glaring at Pat as she approached.

"This poor dumb son of a bitch is gonna bleed to death," he yelled into her face without giving her any information as to what he was talking about. All visitors, security guards, and other staff members froze in place, turning to watch. "And it's all your fault."

"I beg your pardon?" Pat blanched.

He started posturing and screaming. She was able to figure out that he had her mixed up with someone else. There was a time when she would have done whatever she could to rectify the situation anyway. But today she wasn't about to be cowed.

"This man is not my patient," she said calmly, suppressing the desire to match his shouts. "He's not even from my floor. I suggest if you have a problem that you take it up with his attending."

"Who the hell do you think you are?" he demanded. She could see the patient would just as soon inch his covers over his face. "You don't tell me what to do."

"It's not my problem," Pat stated flatly. She turned around and started walking away.

"Get back here, miss," he bellowed. "I haven't dismissed you!"

She ignored him, held her head erect, and kept walking, the security guards applauding as she passed.

She never heard another word from him.

When Judyth sees those kinds of stressors, the first thing that occurs to her is that there are rookies afoot, people who aren't sure about their knowledge and therefore lack confidence. That anxiety leads to a lot of conflicts that the modern world of nursing just hasn't got time for. Judyth has been a nurse for twenty-two years, and in that period has seen the responsibilities of nurses expand enormously. When she graduated from nursing school, she was not permitted to start IVs—this, in a sizable San Francisco teaching institution—or do fluid therapy with medication administration. IV pumps were nonexistent.

With increased technology and the numerous invasive procedures, including heart and lung monitoring, routinely performed by nurses, there is a tremendous amount of pressure on everyone to stay current with the technical aspects of care stages and complexities of healing. Added to that are the pressures of cost-containment DRGs (diagnostic-related groups), which have dramatically increased patient turnaround times from admission to discharge and slashed ancillary staff who used to assist RNs on the floors. To coordinate all the things nurses have to coordinate, there really is not a lot of time left over to interact in a parent-child way with the medical staff.

Peggy, who has worked both staff and supervisory positions in one of the country's foremost trauma centers, believes the nurse-physician dynamic there is almost ideal.

> "There's basically a healthy respect. We get to know each other's skills in depth. It's not uncommon to have a physician say, 'Write whatever orders you need, and I'll co-sign them.' The nurses here have earned that respect. There is a great deal of free rein, and the docs know we'll call them if we have any questions at all."

Learning to establish a flexible relationship with patients is a challenge all new nurses face. In nursing practice, where other human beings are dealt with on the most intimate basis, it is easy to experience an emotional rapport not readily attainable in other occupations. There is always someone seeking a hopeful smile, a merciful eye, a nod of sympathy. Often this is what drew the new nurse into the field; even seasoned nurses maintain it is still the emotional lift they get from direct patient contact that they most prize.

"You really have access to intimacy that's available no other way. That appeals to me. There is an opportunity in a clinical setting to be with a patient in a much more casual, much more intimate way than with someone, say, in a business setting."

When Marguerite worked at Yale, she cared for a forty-three-year-old man named Nick who had an aggressive course of lymphocytic leukemia. Nick was a large man, still muscular despite recurring bouts with various infections to which his illness left him exposed. His hobby before becoming ill had been poling, an uncommon competitive endeavor where one stands in a canoe and pushes it upstream by using long, gondolier-type poles.

Marguerite was working nights when Nick regressed and was transferred to the ICU, beset by yet another dangerous infection. When he returned to the floor, he was on numerous antibiotics that needed to be administered around the clock.

She tried to prepare him for the frequent disturbances. "Well, Nick, looks like I'm gonna have to be in your room every hour or even more often because you've got so many medications."

"Oh, that's fine by me, really. I want you to come in. I'm actually kind of afraid, you know?" He had a clear understanding that he didn't have much time left. "So don't worry about waking me up."

Each time she came in to hang his piggyback IVs or check his vitals, Marguerite gave him a little touch before going out again.

Sometime around dawn, he asked her if she had time to talk.

"You know," he whispered. "Every time you walk in the room, this cool breeze comes in. I really needed somebody to help me get through last night. I just felt so safe because you were here."

It was one of those moments that confirmed the correctness of her choice of career.

The next day, Marguerite worked the evening shift. When she arrived, all the doctors said, "Boy, I'll tell you, he thinks you're just great. He's been telling everybody that an angel was in his room last night. That a divine wind kept blowing into his room, soothing his pain."

When Marguerite went into his room, Nick gave her a plant he'd had his wife bring as a gift for her.

A week later, when leaving for the night, she told him, "Well, you take care now, Nick. You know I'm not gonna be back till midnight tomorrow night, so I'll stop in and see you as soon as I'm here."

The next night, she arrived a little early for her shift. As soon as she came in, the charge nurse told her, "He's been asking all shift when you'd get here. You'd better get in there quick if you want to see him. We think he's dying."

Nick's family was in the room sitting with him, faces strained and teary or stony. He was still alive, looking markedly more frail than even the day before. His wife introduced her affectionately to her children as Daddy's divine wind. She later nominated Marguerite for Connecticut's Cancer Nurse of the Year.

"I've been waiting for you," he murmured.

"I know," she said, taking a seat and holding his hand. "Thank you, Nick."

His wife held his other hand. A few minutes later, he died.

Marguerite still has the card Nick gave her with the plant, one of a small treasured collection: *For my divine wind. Thanks for getting me through the night, Nick.*

The commitment to patients usually takes a toll. Most nurses have to deal with *the savior syndrome* at some time. Barbara was the nurse for a male patient, Phil, admitted for repeat bypass surgery. She had been Phil's nurse for his first operation and had developed a deep, reciprocal caring for both him and his wife, Alice. Phil didn't make it through his second surgery. The night he died, Barbara sat with Alice, consoling her, doing whatever she could to comfort her. Barbara didn't care if that hospital burned down around them—she wasn't leaving Alice's side as long as she needed her.

Committed as she was, Barbara realized she couldn't do this all the time. It was too draining. She was exhausted afterward, her concentration spoiled for other patients and her own life. She started distancing herself emotionally from her patients, inspiring concerns about becoming too mechanical in her work. Over time she found a way to be concerned about patients without allowing it to turn into hurt. There have been some since who have cut through to her heart, but they have been fewer.

The problem of confronting the sobering shortcomings of humanity becomes known to all new nurses. Eventually, there is a challenge to any value system the nurse carries into the job. If not encountered in school, the unsavoriness of human behavior will surely be met in the first months of practice: the boy who blows his nose in the bed sheets so he can have a laugh when the nurse arrives to straighten them, bringing up a handful of mucus; the man with a GI bleed—and GI bleeds have probably the most intense sickly odor—who swaggers naked down the hall, scratching his scrotum swaying between his knees, spitting out bloody clots while yelling, "Gimme a beer! Gimme a beer!"

Forget racial, ethnic, and cultural differences, to which nursing students are instructed to be sensitive—the behaviors of some patients seem to place them in another species.

A nursing function heavily stressed in school is that of being the *patient advocate*. It means that the nurse is supposed to help patients understand the system, using it to their advantage, and intercede on the patient's behalf if problems arise with other health professionals. It also means making sure respect is accorded and rights safeguarded, even to the point of refusing a physician's order if it is thought to be not in the patient's best interest.

In that regard, Doris once participated in what she thought of as a bizarre incident. She was working in an ICU when a woman was admitted after being badly beaten by her boyfriend. She had a broken femur, fem-pop (femoral-popliteal, two arteries in the leg) bypasses, nose and cheek fractures. He'd really done a job on her.

During the assault, however, she'd killed the guy—shot him or stabbed him, something appropriate to his behavior. The cops were in questioning her, a guard sitting by the door.

An outside observer might conclude, Good riddance to bad trash. The creep got what he deserved. That certainly was how most of the nursing staff felt. But when she regained consciousness, she was remorseful and self-hating, mourning her man. At one point, she wanted to kill herself, pulling out her IVs and tearing at her dressings.

"I don't care. I don't care!" she shrieked and wept. "I want to be with him."

She wound up in restraints, had a psych consult, the whole nine yards.

She kept trying to convince the psychiatrist that she should be permitted to leave the hospital to attend the viewing to mourn her loss. And the psychiatrist was leaning toward letting her go when Doris and the other staff nurses convinced him it would be counter-therapeutic, to put it mildly. Not only was she unable to display any measurable degree of self-control, in and out of restraints, but they had also been informed that some of the boyfriend's family members were inclined to take up where he'd left off if they could get their hands on her.

Ultimately, a compromise was worked out where the boyfriend's body could be brought to the hospital, after visiting hours, for an open-casket viewing. The mortician set up the lobby with flowers just like a funeral home. Doris arranged the whole thing with the undertaker, administration, security, the woman's family, and the family of the deceased. Luckily, his mother was sympathetic.

A couple of psychiatric technicians were recruited from the

psych unit to accompany the patient down to the lobby for her own mini-wake. All this so that she could "resolve her grief."

One of the techs who helped transport her had a boom box with music she'd requested: "You Were Always On My Mind." For a while that became the unit theme song. Humming it was a way of quietly commenting about particularly hateful patients.

It doesn't take long to start questioning the limits of caring.

> "You get a feeling of being used and abused a bit. But I think that's just nursing. Some of the things nurses do with people are so intimate, so distasteful to the person—I mean, we're talking about wiping people's behinds for them, cleaning up their vomit, seeing them in states more helpless than anything since they were infants—that patients sometimes dehumanize us in order to be able to cope with us. That isn't always the nicest thing in the world. Sometimes my anger would flare because of that."

Nurses talk about the *burnout cycle*: The graduate nurse is finally out of school, eager for experience, open to challenge. The first six months are very exciting, a lot of learning and growth occur, she is very up. Then she gets singed a time or two—maybe deep-fry charred—by patients or administration, by the doctors, by other nurses.

Guilt can begin to flow from the work and follow nurses into their private lives. Early in her career, Karen went on a ski trip with some friends. Somebody on the bus made a crack about hospitals being death houses even if entered for a broken bone.

"Oh, that's not true," she said blithely. "We cure'm all."

"Not my uncle," said the guy in the seat behind her, his tone angrily pointed. "He died."

She felt he blamed her.

Another time, she was in a funeral home for a great-aunt who'd died an unexpected death. There was an older lady there who looked familiar but whom Karen couldn't place. She approached her and asked if they had met before. The woman burst into tears.

"You were one of the nurses who took care of my husband," the woman gasped. "And he's dead!"

"I felt horrible. I couldn't remember his name or what he had, but I could recall which bed he'd been in."

New nurses often retreat, a layer of protective cynicism starting to grow. Lines start to be drawn between *us* and *them*. Labeling others becomes a common buffer. Acronyms and gallows humor abound: "If it isn't documented, it can't be traced to you. . . ." "If you can't treat the patient, treat the chart." Physicians become "CYOA (cover your own ass) certified." Patients are known by bed numbers or diagnosis, both genuine—"the hernia in '81-B"—and improvised—"PPP" (piss poor protoplasm), "LOLINAD" (little old lady in no apparent distress), "BOD" (better off dead), "the 3Bs" (brain dead, but breathing), and the ever-popular, all-purpose "GOMER" (get out of my emergency room).

In the best circumstances, there are buffers built into the system, a period of orientation. Traditionally this lasts a minimum of several weeks, allowing new nurses to become acquainted with guideline policies and procedures, the layout of the physical plant and departmental hierarchies, accessing fax machines and computer terminals.

In smaller hospitals, orientation is usually given by the head nurse on the floor. Larger institutions often employ staff development educators, clinical specialists, or senior staff preceptors—RN resource people theoretically in less authoritarian, more approachable positions—to ease the transition into the real world. Preceptors focus on clinical adjustments, reinforcing time management and prioritization skills learned in school, helping pinpoint strengths and weaknesses, and sorting out chain-of-command delegation problems. They may also help reconcile new nurses with the emotional overload of the work.

Very often, though, transitions are quite abrupt and unsupported.

Anna started her career at a university-affiliated, statewide referral hospital in West Virginia. Because she wanted to avail herself of educational benefits, she wound up working the night shift and taking classes during the day. She and another nurse, both new grads, ran a fifty-bed floor with an LPN and two aides. Patients who were exceptionally difficult cases, who had overwhelmed the abilities of their local hospitals, were sent there from all over the state. What she was unable to appreciate at the time, lacking experience for comparison, was that the majority of patients on general floors in that institution would have been in intensive care units in any other hospital.

There were patients in frank pulmonary edema from congestive heart failure (CHF), the heart unable to expel enough blood to meet the body's needs, huffing and gurgling with their feet down to pool blood. Nurses were giving "IV push" Lasix (a powerful diuretic), which hospital policy limited to administration by physicians but the supervisors had said was acceptable practice. There were people with chest tubes draining, people on ventilators. . . .

Initially, Anna assumed that the degree of difficulty she encountered was due to her newness in the profession, that she needed to improve her skills to keep from running behind, to learn to prioritize and budget her time better. Her head nurse was certainly willing to support this perspective. Anna was always running behind, playing catch up. It was always, "Hurry, hurry, hurry!" "Move, move, move!" Everybody had more than they could handle. There wasn't even time to orient new staff to policies and procedures or simply where supplies were kept and staff toilets located. New faces were pointed toward the hallway with a list of bed numbers they were responsible for.

"When I was very new, it used to bother me to find someone dead in bed. The first time that happened, I recall putting my head down on the steering wheel and sobbing in the parking lot after the shift. It would still upset me, but I now know that the problems at the hospital were because of the institution itself and not my fault. There were just too many people for two new grads to adequately care for. You couldn't be all the places you needed to be."

She remained for eight months. By then it had become too grim. She was one of a hundred nurses who resigned by the end of that time. Whole floors, whole services were shut down. A staffing crisis developed as people left and were not replaced. Those who remained felt punished for being there because it was so horrendous. More people routinely called in sick, thereby adding again to the load of those who showed up, grinding down their ability to even face the work, much less perform it.

It's not unusual for new nurses to be plunged into extreme life-and-death circumstances requiring immediate action right from the start. Doris had been out of school only a brief time when she was working evenings on a floor where each wing had thirty-two patients covered by a single RN and an aide. The usual routine was that whoever got her own work done first went down the hall to see if she could help her friends. No one was ever left alone; always as a group. If it meant staying until 2:00 A.M. to get caught up—and there were always things to be caught up on—so be it.

"That's the most unbelievable part of it to me today. We were all so new, we didn't even question it. Still, I enjoyed it. We became very close to one another, as people and professionals."

An obese female patient, Frannie, in her forties and in for a fractured hip, had been requesting all shift for staff to get her out of bed to have a bowel movement, insisting she could not use a bedpan. At about 10:00 P.M., everything else being done,

Doris decided it was time to help this woman out of bed. She called together "the bod squad," and Fran was carefully transferred to a wheelchair with much angling and dangling, strain, sweat, and several, "Okay, on the count of three" commands. The bathroom was barely big enough for the patient alone, much less the two nurses able to squeeze in to assist her onto the toilet.

They stepped outside to give her some privacy and themselves a breather, stretching backs and wiping brows. A minute later Fran let out a yelp.

"Are you okay?" Doris cracked the door to check on her. She found the woman clutching at her breast, wheezing, face pale and grimacing, half-slumped, contorted on the toilet. The woman went rigid and slumped against the wall. Doris crouched before her, feeling for a pulse and finding none.

"Oh, my God, call a code!"

She wedged into the room, scrambling around limbs and trying to get a grip, needing to get Frannie to the floor to start CPR. The nurse accompanying Doris later told her that she had screamed for help at the top of her lungs, but Doris had no memory of that, no memory of the PA system Code Blue call transmitted overhead. She remembers only the repeated phrase, spoken or not, "Oh, shit! Oh, shit!" and the cold terror in her heart.

Doris made the decision, The hell with her hip, dipped at the knees, hoisted and angled Fran toward the door, inching outward for what seemed like hours, steps as tiny and tentative as a golfer at his tee, fecal stains smearing the front of her uniform. There had been nothing like this in Nursing 101. On the floor in the doorway, still cramped, they dragged her across the floor into the hallway, where there was room to begin resuscitation. Doris doesn't recall the clattering of crash-cart wheels arriving or the teams of racing feet, only kneeling over this dying woman, praying with each compression, "Oh, God, get me *out* of here! Why did I ever go into this kind of work?"

Helping new staff members come to grips with the necessary invasions of another person's body and the unavoidable loss of some life was a challenge to Sharan when a head nurse. She tended to see the over-involvement in younger staff nurses, those who called in on their free time to check on their patients, those who extended their shifts unreasonably, especially if they weren't looking for overtime. They needed more counseling in the areas of stress management, refocusing and letting go when patients were lost—and not feeling inadequate or uncaring if they did so—not getting caught up in the painful moment, the family's grief, becoming dysfunctional. They had to focus on those patients who still needed them.

Most patients were trauma victims—basically healthy, if severely injured, people. The majority were young, easy for new nurses to identify with: this one reminds you of your brother, that one your son; ''I'm the same age and background as her. . . .'' It took its toll.

For Sharan, the most successful nurses are those able to separate and leave the work at work. The nurses able to do so were the ones with another focus in their lives. They were married, they had children, they were in school, or they had a consuming hobby. She strongly encouraged her nurses to take their vacations and time off, to switch hats and involve themselves in healthy outside pursuits.

> ''Letting go doesn't mean that if you lose a patient, if a patient dies, that you don't grieve for that person. You do. I've grieved for every patient I've lost. But you have to compartmentalize: 'I've got this to do now, and then I have to cover that problem for that patient. . . . I'll grieve when I'm finished. . . .'
>
> ''You learn to do that. Or you don't survive. Part of it just comes with maturity and experience within the nursing profession.''

Most new nurses spend the first year or two solidifying skills and adapting to the limits of the system. Ideals are tarnished, if still intact. They have experienced the crunch of being in a position of extraordinary responsibility with little authority, and adapted their private expectations to reality.

Lena's first position was the night shift on a med-surg research floor in a large urban hospital, one of two nurses responsible for twenty-six to thirty patients. There were supposed to be two nurse's aides also, but more than half the time there was only one. In the beginning, it was very frustrating, being expected to care for too many patients, doing too many things with too little experience, and feeling like she couldn't do a good enough job. These were acutely medically ill people, mostly MA (medical assistance) and street people.

Many of the patients had CHF, hepatitis, or AIDS. Many were alcoholics, many drug addicts with sepsis: people who had no intention of altering the behaviors that led to hospitalization. Chronicity is something that is read about in school but is never really experienced because clinical time is so brief. In the workplace, it's not just a matter of sending them out the door and waving good-bye. They come back. And some of them keep coming back. The first reaction is often anger—perhaps shielding a deeper sense of guilt: "Maybe I didn't do a good enough job"—growing into cynicism with the numbness of repetition: "Christ, I already know his story. . . . Let's see how he's screwed up *this* time."

Lena felt her schooling had prepared her as best it could for clinical situations, but this was just a whole new ball game. There were many arrests, many deaths. She felt like she was barely treading water. When she first learned there was an AIDS patient on the floor, she was very apprehensive about being assigned to him. When she was, she became extremely cautious, gowning and double gloving for every procedure, wiping her hands with alcohol afterward, going home the first time and washing her uniform twice, showering twice.

Eventually she got to thinking, "Well, you either need to adjust to this or leave. You just can't go on this way."

She started observing how other people went in and out of

the room without extreme precautions. Clearly, some people were more comfortable with it than others. She reacquainted herself with proper procedures and started learning more about it.

Gradually it became less worrisome.

After twelve to eighteen months, the new nurse is no longer new. Questions about career direction begin to surface. Many hit a point where they ask themselves, "Is this all there is?" They start looking for a way to advance themselves and either make a job change or get out altogether, some to other careers, some returning to school for other areas within the profession. Most settle in for the long haul, hoping that their head nurse will get married, move away, or evaporate so they can take her job and get to follow the Monday through Friday, 8:00 A.M. to 4:30 P.M. schedule around which the civilian world rotates.

Cathy found she needed to move on in order to be able to function at the level she felt capable of attaining. Her first experience was in an affluent suburban Chicago hospital. Despite being a straight A student, she found it overwhelming. Mostly she was frightened, feeling she was more a danger than a help to patients in that first year. While some new nurses she knew seemed to grasp things immediately, almost inately knowing how to handle any situation, she thinks most were struggling as hard as she.

Self-confidence came through seeing everything once and learning, through mistakes she made, how to handle situations the second time around. Eventually, it all started to click and come together. That took about a year and a half. By then she knew it was time to change hospitals. It was necessary to leave in order to break out of the image of "the fumbling new grad" held by her head nurse and co-workers, who were relentless with reminders of mistakes made in greener days.

Peggy, on the other hand, hating change of any kind, preferred to stay where she started, working her entire eighteen-year career in one of the largest trauma centers in the country.

In the beginning, it was still a relatively small facility, very much a mom-and-pop organization. When she was hired, Peggy had an interview with the nursing director, which is a rarity, such tasks usually falling to head nurses, nurse recruiters, or one of several assistant directors.

Peggy came from a strong Italian family background, and the hospital became a second home for her. The medical director was very much a father figure and the director of nursing a strong maternal force. Looking back, she can see there was definite substitution occurring. Her father died while she was still in orientation, galvanizing her desire to help people, to make it better for others because she couldn't make it better for him.

The hospital was quite willing to put that energy to use. The standard assumption at that time was to be institute-oriented. When she interviewed Peggy, the director of nursing had a cot in her office where she could nap. She hadn't gone home in sixteen days. It was a place where people gave of themselves. The medical director had a cot in his office also. There was a sense of dedication one feels for a family. Nurses were praised for working unpaid overtime and praised for volunteering to do anything that was needed. Peggy recalls remaining on duty once for thirty-six hours so that a unit could remain open. She did it because the director of nursing, solely on the power of her relationship with Peggy, asked her to.

The way Peggy deals with job stress and frustration is to switch units and speciality areas every few years. Each position offers its own new experiences, rewards, defeats, and surprises. She was one of the first to work in the admitting area when it was a new unit. That was in '73, her first such inter-unit transition.

The essential difference between an emergency room and a trauma admitting unit is that of speed and treatment availability. In a trauma center, appropriate equipment and staff are immediately available. A traumatologist is in the house at all times. Likewise an anesthesiologist, an OR team, a thoracic surgeon.

General hospital staffs decrease to a skeleton crew on weekends, nights, and holidays, the busiest times for trauma. Unless trauma happens on a weekday, nine to five, most of those people are at home on call. Precious time needed to reverse the shock process is wasted.

Peggy transferred to the admitting area from the intensive care unit, needing a change of pace, new challenges. There was variability in the schedule, which she found refreshing, downtime between patients taken up with blessedly mindless tasks like putting surgical trays back together, stocking supplies before the next bout of focused frenzy in stabilizing shock candidates. If there was absolutely nothing to do, she would drift back to one of the critical care units to help out, a beeper on a belt to announce arrivals.

It was a nice change, not always having a patient on her mind. As an ICU nurse, she had primary care patients whose condition she was responsible for from admission to discharge—writing their care plans, setting up social service contacts and aftercare follow-ups, and moderating family conferences. They occupied a place in her mind whether she was working or at home. In the admitting area, there was that intensity of effort to stabilize someone, but then the patient was quickly shipped out to the OR or an ICU.

Peggy was the first nurse in the admitting area when the alert came for a double admission, two young girls arriving via ambulance. . . .

Their mother, Rachel, jokingly called her girls her New Frontier Family. The oldest, Kelly, was born in the snowbank winter of '61, just after JFK's inauguration. It was a hopeful time for a young couple finishing college—he law, she psychology—to start a family, but Bernadette was born in darker days, and Rachel was pregnant with Amy when news of Kennedy's assassination was broadcast. They huddled on their couch, babies nearby, touching them often; they couldn't bear to have them out of reach. Rachel never guessed how painful the desire to protect could be. There was a war in Southeast Asia; there were lynchings in the South. And now this. Something was pulling apart in America. There was no sleeping. They rocked and wept and were glued to the TV.

Kelly, twelve, excelled in gymnastics and track-and-field. She studied ballet at her mother's insistence but thought it really dopey. Bernadette agreed. Graceless and already outgrowing her older sister, she was developing a strain of sarcasm that she often employed on the family, even referring to her mother by her first name, though rarely to her face.

That day, Kelly and Bernie walked the two suburban blocks to fetch hamburger buns from the 7-Eleven for dinner. They were crossing the two-lane road, slick from a summer afternoon shower, when the tractor trailer rounded the bend. Air brakes hissed, too late. The sisters clutched each other and were hit. There were no eyewitnesses, just those who came running after the impact and screech of tires.

Rachel wasn't worried about their tardiness. Lately they were always at each other, jostling and chasing and putting each other down. She later recalled hearing sirens a few blocks off, but it wasn't an uncommon sound and caused her no concern. She had a small TV on the kitchen countertop and was chopping vegetables absently, engrossed in watching the Watergate hearings. For the first time in a decade, things seemed to be righting themselves.

Then a boy from the junior high was pounding on her door.

The trauma team formed as the ambulances arrived, separating to work on the broken bodies. They were brought in strapped to body boards, laid out on trauma tables ten feet apart. They had multiple fractures, lacerations, sucking chest wounds. The team was fighting time, fighting failure. In those days, it was policy that no one was ever pronounced dead on arrival. Everyone was taken in and worked on—blood poured back into them, chests cracked to see if something could be fixed.

Still, they immediately recognized the unlikelihood of survival. Agreeing that there was no hope for the slender girl—light hair browned by blood and soot, EKG barely fluttering, left leg almost severed, probable spinal damage—they concentrated on the darker, larger one, telling themselves she might have a chance.

"We've got to save *one* of these girls," someone said.

Peggy remained with the slender child, latex gloves slick with her blood, checking for absent pupil reaction, respirations irregularly irregular—"Biot's breaths," probably from increased intracranial pressure. Her pulse pressure was sluggish, thinning to nil, her child's heart exhausted. At the very end, Peggy removed a glove and touched her, sliding her mask down, inching up to her ear.

"You're not alone, sweetheart," she whispered, smelling the faintest scent of baby powder on her neck. "You're not alone. I'm gonna stay right here with you."

Her body was removed to the morgue while the team made what repairs they could on her sister, who was ready to be whooshed away to the OR. The elevator waited, transport techs readied for the run. IV tubing swayed like bunting in a breeze, and she was gone, two minutes door to door, and God help any idiot who wandered into their path. Potential trauma everywhere.

Blood and treatment debris were all that remained. They busied themselves cleaning, readying. No one wanted to speak, to say what everyone knew: she wouldn't make it either. Not a chance. The traumatologist was steeling himself to speak with the family when a call for another admission came.

"Oh, jeez," he sighed, wiping his face, checking his watch, and glancing around the room. "Peg, I need you to do me a favor. . . ."

She stripped off her surgical gown, disposed of gloves, nodding, knowing the family needed to be told something.

He nodded back, shrugging helplessly.

"Tell them . . . jeez, I dunno—they need to be prepared for this." He made a slow sweeping gesture around the room. "Just tell'm that they're not doing real well. . . . That I'll be down to speak with them as soon as I can. Okay?"

Working as an emergency-room-unit clerk while in nursing school, Peggy had seen others take this walk. She had admired the doctors and nurses who performed this task of the telling. She always knew she'd get her turn but never realized how difficult this news could be to convey.

She walked down the corridor deliberately, with a stiffened pace, left foot following right, overhearing a senseless dispute with a security guard ("That damn vending machine kept my quarter!"), drying her palms on her hips, her left hand rising to pull the door open, explanations forming, a buffer of phrases: all that can be done is being done; where there's life, there's hope; it happened so fast, I'm sure she didn't suffer.

She entered the family waiting room. The remaining family sat on the couch, the youngest daughter between her parents, folded over, elbows on knees, shredding tissue swaths that gathered about her bare feet. Three tearful faces froze upward expectantly at the click of the door. Peggy introduced herself flatly, feeling the catch of tears in her voice, her throat too dry to swallow.

Scanning them, she caught the mother's eyes. In the pause that followed, Rachel said, "They're dead, aren't they?"

The sustaining illusion of hope was sucked away as if by a punch. Suppressed sobs choked Peggy.

"Yeah," was all she could respond.

Rachel extended her hand, and Peggy took it. This woman's dying daughter was the last person Peggy had touched.

"Both of them?"

"Well." Peggy nodded. "Truthfully, yes."

The father was hugging his remaining child, both in tears. Peggy tried to stifle her own sobbing.

"They were dead when we left," Rachel said softly. "We knew that."

"I'm so sorry," Peggy sobbed. She sat in the chair beside Rachel, who inched forward, each on the edge of her seat, knees touching, fingers clasping, sharing the piercing loss.

"We did all we could."

"I know you did. I know."

They rocked together, hugging. It took several minutes before she began feeling unprofessional, out of control, as if the mother was helping *her* deal with the tragedy.

"I'll have the doctor come down and tell you just exactly what the injuries were."

"It doesn't matter now."

"She smelled like baby powder. . . ." Peggy said, wanting to offer something.

"Kelly," Rachel whispered, identifying the child for Peggy. "Do you have a minute? Can I tell you a little about them?"

"Yes. Please do."

Rachel told her all about her family while her husband rocked and wept, and Peggy pulled herself together. They held hands so hard it hurt.

Afterward, Peggy returned to the admitting area, her hatred of the doctor growing with each step. He was sitting in the lounge when she found him, smoking, writing up the second admission.

"Hard, huh?" he asked, seeing her face.

"Why did you do that to me?" she demanded. "*How* could you do that to me?"

He stood and crossed the room to her.

"Because I knew you would go down there and that you'd be the most sensitive person for them. Because I respect you, Peg. I knew there was another admission coming in, and I had to stay fresh for the one who might still be alive. I had to keep my edge and stay prepared. I really trusted that you could handle it."

"At the time, I just wanted to give him a furious whipping. Now I know that what he did was okay. I now know that a lot of the grief I felt about my father's death was all mixed in there. It certainly helped speed up my own grieving process. It was something I had to get used to dealing with. This was my chosen profession."

4

"All That Can Be Done"

The Emergency Room

The hospital hums. The sound, coming from huge air-conditioning units on the roof, drifts out over the neighborhood like a muffled dentist's drill. The hospital fills a single city square. The original building is seven stories high, a blunt red-brick rectangle. Additional wings of orange brick face, chevroning off the east and west tail sections, have been added over the years. Still, it is small by the standards of modern medical centers with an inpatient capacity of just over 250.

It was founded by a religious order of nursing nuns around the turn of the century. At that time, the surrounding area was suburban, even rural. The wealth and care of that era can still be glimpsed in ornamental details of some of the older buildings. Since then, the city has swelled, becoming one of the five largest in the country. Today the neighborhood is mostly concrete, congestion, and urban decay.

In America today, there are approximately 7,000 hospitals. The National Association for Hospital Development, however, estimates that by the year 2000, only 4,100 will survive. Between 1988 and 1990, two hundred acute-care facilities failed. This is just the kind of institution that is expected to go under—a nonprofit, inner-city general community hospital providing basic health services to a population of over 200,000. The hospital is already operating in the red. Funding comes largely in the form of public assistance. Many patients have no health insurance at all. There is a high degree of chronic illness and poor compliance with medical recommendations. Illiteracy, drug abuse, alcoholism, teenage pregnancy, and fragmented home situations—all the things that are the cause and effect of poverty—are rampant. That is baseline. It has been estimated that one of every four males between the ages of thirteen and twenty-five in this neighborhood will die violently in drug-, gang-, or family-related conflicts.

Mary Beth, who worked in the ICU for several years, describes it this way:

> "In this hospital, the people you see are already so down-trodden, they already have total body failure. You're trying to patch up one aspect, but you can forget it. . . . They are never going to be optimum. There's not a whole lot of self-actualization going on here. Just people destroying themselves with the same old shit—drugs, alcohol, stabbings, and gunshots to the here, there, and everywhere . . . Seems like you patch'm up and then next month or next year, they're back. It gets so you recognize old surgical scars: 'Hey, didn't Dr. G. sew this up here last year?'
>
> "You get these cocky young guys with their gunshot wounds as trophies. They're just aching to go out and get the next one. They love to call you 'bitch!' If you had your own gun, it would be tempting to shoot the little mothers yourself.
>
> "Hospitals acquire reputations. The word on this institution is that if you are in need of admission to a medical floor, go elsewhere or stay at home. This isn't someplace that's high on the choice list for medical schools. Nobody's coming here to do ground-breaking research. But if you're ever shot or in an auto accident, the ER here is the place to go. Blunt and penetrating trauma—that's our speciality. . . . *C'mon down!*"

Being an emergency-department triage nurse is an exercise in uncertainty, each shift a roll of the dice as to how active it will be, what tragedy will arrive at the door. Contrary to health care mythology, there is no real pattern to arrivals. The usually cited times—an hour after the bars close, full moons, holiday dinners when the family fun turns mean—can pass as peacefully as a Sunday brunch, while a midweek afternoon can explode with the skirl of sirens and the intercom call for assistance: "TRAUMA ALERT IN THE EMERGENCY DEPARTMENT . . . ! REPEAT—EMERGENCY DEPARTMENT TRAUMA ALERT!"

It has been Kathleen's job since 1985.

"While the ER has more flexibility than the floors, it's also scarier. You never get to the point where you feel entirely proficient. I have books I buy, I just signed up for a conference in pediatric trauma, but I still don't feel proficient. I know that as far as basic skills are concerned, I'm a very good nurse, but like for snap decisions . . . it can get hairy.

"You can be certified in this and that, you can be reading all you can and there will always be that one thing—an impalement of the eye or something you haven't a clue what to do with—and you're praying somebody else knows more about it than you do. When that happens, you thank God if there's another nurse there who has dealt with it or something similar before.

"Still, you're always afraid of that time when you're the most experienced nurse there. It has happened to me, and it can be terrifying."

Working in the emergency department was not Kathleen's first choice. She had been working in the medical intensive care unit (MICU) only a few months when the administration decided it was necessary to close the unit. Adequate numbers of RNs could not be found to staff it. It was the onset of the nursing shortage. Kathleen had a choice: either transfer to the ER or go to a floor known to staff as the Cabbage Patch—all respirators and people who wanted cigarettes while on vents. People who smoked through the tracheostomy holes in their necks.

The ER won out.

Another incentive in coming to the ER was being able to take advantage of a special program allowing RNs to work weekends only, a twelve-hour shift every Saturday and Sunday, while receiving the same pay and benefits as full-time, day-shift employees. As a mother of two, Kathleen was afforded maximum time for her family. The actual title of the program is the Baylor Plan, but it is known more broadly as the "weekend option," or simply "twelve to twelve." It was a recruitment and retention strategy introduced during the last nursing shortage—in the late seventies and early eighties—to help stabilize nursing staffs. As a special program, it may be terminated by administrative fiat at any time without getting into sticky labor-relations problems. Most hospitals originally using it did away with it as soon as there was a glut in the pool of available RNs in the early 1980s.

(Kathleen's hospital retained the program, believing it a cheaper alternative to being bled by prices paid out to private nursing agencies in order to keep units open. Agencies pay more per hour than hospitals, benefit outlays converted directly into cash. On top of the hourly rate, a fee is also paid to the agency, making it an expensive proposition. The agency responsible for running New York City's eleven public hospitals had outlays in the neighborhood of $60 million for agency nurses in 1989.)

At first, the program was limited to speciality areas—intensive care units, OR, ER; areas where the shortages were first obvious—but as the shortage stain spread to taint all aspects of health care, it was expanded to include the entire institution. There was already an active "nursing pool" in house. Pools are another tool devised by hospitals to combat the expense of agencies. Nurses who already work for a hospital may pick up extra "pool time." While they are paid the same as agency nurses, the additional agency fee is forgone and, because pool nurses are familiar with hospital policies, procedures, and physical layout, precious time is not squandered on orientation. Pools also allow hospitals to cut down on paying overtime to fill schedule vacancies.

The topic of such flexibility in schedules is a prickly issue among some nurses, often portrayed as an example of fragmented care impacting negatively upon patients. It's not an argument Kathleen entirely buys. Back when she started, nurses had their schedules made up three weeks in advance. Within that period, she worked all three shifts. And it was never consistent; she might do two days of day shift, followed by an evening shift leading into a night shift, then a day off only to return on a day shift. There wasn't a whole lot of concern from the administration in those days about how exhaustion affected patient care. It's just that with the shortage, staff nurses are in a stronger market position to dictate better arrangements for themselves. For the first time, administrations are the ones that have to be flexible.

Though she has been in nursing since 1973, usually full-time, Kathleen doesn't consider herself a career nurse. She works because she needs the money. It's an attitude she attributes to her experience with nursing administrations in general, and a previous director of nursing (DON) in particular. When the hospital started its pool, Kathleen was working on the full-time ICU staff, often pulling charge duty on nights, making just over nine dollars hourly; that with four years experience and sequentially good work evaluations. She took a leave of absence to have her second child, planning to return.

The DON called her after a few weeks, inquiring about her plans.

Kathleen mentioned to her that the nurses who worked in the pool were making almost five dollars more an hour. Here she was, loyal on staff, not deserting to the pool, taking on charge responsibilities, and feeling that in order to justify returning to that slot . . . well, she thought maybe she'd need ten dollars an hour.

There was a tense silence before the DON curtly said, "I have to tell you, Kathleen, I'm more than a little insulted. Your job is here if you want to come back to it, but you'll come back at the rate you left at. You're on maternity leave, so you won't lose your benefits, but *that's* it.''

"I think I should tell you,'' Kathleen responded, more than a little insulted herself, "that I've heard about what other hospitals are paying. As a matter of fact, I've spoken with two other recruiters over the phone. They don't even know me or my work, much less my good performance evaluations, but they're willing to start me at ten an hour, sight unseen. Plus, they're suburban hospitals, so there's no city-wage tax withheld there.''

"Kathleen, I'm shocked,'' the DON said. Kathleen could almost swear she felt the frost come through the phone. "That is so disloyal. You have no right to shop around like that. There are patients here who depend upon you.''

"I beg your pardon.'' Kathleen mustered her courage, partly guilty in her soul because she *did* feel disloyal, having been socialized in nursing school to consider the hospital almost an extension of the family. Administrators have made an art out of making staff members feel as if any decision made in self-interest immediately endangers the lives of patients. "But I've got to put bread and butter on my table, and I *do* have the right to shop around anywhere and anytime I see fit. If you can't see a way to give me a raise—especially since I've never had a single merit increase for my good evaluations—then we're at an impasse. I'm asking you to renegotiate a wage for me that's acceptable so I don't have to have an argument with my husband, who knows what I've been offered elsewhere. He's in a world where he gets raises left and right, and he can't understand this having to beg.''

"Kathleen, you've heard my terms.''

Kathleen resigned as a full-time staff nurse and went into the pool, in the very same hospital, making an extra five dollars per hour. But she felt bad about it. It wasn't what she'd wanted, preferring to be on a single unit, to take charge and keep learning in an area of interest. In the pool, she was bounced from unit to unit, losing a sense of continuity of care.

Over time she adapted, doing the best she could in the time allotted and letting that be enough. The paychecks helped, too.

Remembering the guilty aches, she could only think, Boy, were you nuts.

ER patients rarely arrive in an orderly progression. The norm is for lengthy lulls punctuated by waves of the ill and infirm washing up at the door. Treatment gridlock is a common occurrence. Kathleen has passed entire shifts wading through the waiting room sorting and reshuffling triage priorities. ER triage is simpler than military triage. In the ER, the sickest or most damaged patients take precedence, bumping those already waiting down the list.

On her last shift, a woman stayed with her daughter for over two hours awaiting the results of cranial X rays. The little girl had been in a minor auto accident. There had been profuse bleeding, common in scalp injuries, which was medically inconsequential but terrifying to the child and her mother. The bleeding had long ceased, her wound cleansed and bandaged by her nurse, and her neuro-checks were normal. However, they had been seen only once, briefly, by the physician, and were eager for results.

Unfortunately, soon after they were settled in one of the dozen curtained cubicles, a succession of six rescue wagons had arrived within the span of twenty minutes. Three were motor accidents, two very serious, heads through windshields, multiple lacerations. The other three were an overdose and two asthmatics, each acutely compromised. The staff had all they could handle just to keep hopping from one patient to the next.

The mother, anger sprouting from her anxiety, began pacing the hall, purposefully obstructing staff at times, reminding anyone who would listen that she was "*still* waiting!" and making it very clear that she did not appreciate being bumped as a priority.

The third time she stuck her head into the triage room, Kathleen interrupted the physical exam of her patient and stepped into the hall to confer with her, planting her ample frame in the door to afford the partially disrobed patient behind her some privacy.

"Mrs. W., I know it's frustrating to wait. . . ." She began her practiced homily, digging her hands into the pockets of her floral-patterned smock. "And believe me, I don't mean to be callous—I know it was a terrifying experience—but your daughter's wounds were not serious. . . ."

"Oh," Mrs. W. interrupted sarcastically. "And are *you* a doctor?"

It's a line as old as salt; every nurse has heard it.

"It's like I told you before." Kathleen swallowed her irritation. "The doctor will be with you as soon as he can."

"And when's that gonna be? I haven't even seen him go by for a half hour. What is it, dinnertime?"

Tears and groans were clearly audible from the last cubicle on the left.

"Actually, right now, he's sewing up someone's scalp. It was a very bad case. . . ."

"Yeah?" Mrs. W., hands on hips, interrogated with a bitchy tone. "And what happens if he gets a *dozen* bad cases all at once?"

"I'll tell you what happens, Mrs. W." Kathleen exhaled deeply, shaking back her dark, shoulder-length hair, wondering if she'd be reported, written up, and reprimanded, but at the moment not caring in the least. "They've got some damn good-ass nurses watching them who know what to do to help until a doctor *can* get to them!"

Emergency department staffing usually consists of two physicians, five nurses, a unit clerk, and a nurse's aide. ER physicians usually wear scrubs or a lab coat atop street clothes and, if male, a tie. ER nurses' uniforms are varied. Few wear white, most donning a blue surgical scrub suit with the hospital logo imprinted on the breast pocket, a stethoscope slung around the neck. Some wear an overall-type outfit with extra pockets for handy accessories—tape, scissors, tourniquets, gloves, alcohol swatches. Since AIDS arrived, face masks, goggles, and ankle-length OR coats are becoming customary.

AIDS anxiety is present among most health care workers and is of keen concern to ER personnel. Unexpected exposure to the blood and body fluids of unknown individuals is a common experience there. Several of the earliest and most publicized cases of health care workers who became infected through needle sticks or blood splashes were in emergency departments. There is wide variation in estimates of the number of health workers who have been infected while on the job. By late 1991, the Center for Disease Control (CDC) was acknowledging a minimum of sixty cases (up from sixteen, two years before) while speculating the figure may be well over one hundred. Others double that figure. In 1990, at least eighteen lawsuits were pending by employees against hospitals because of job-related HIV infections.

Interestingly, the apprehension associated with exposure has not always translated into action. A study conducted at the Johns Hopkins Hospital ER observed personnel for thirty-one days. Findings demonstrated that in the most likely situations for exposure to the virus—major trauma with profuse bleeding—protective barriers like those mentioned above are least likely to be employed. Despite extensive education and the belief that such barriers could protect them, staff cited the pressure of emergency situations, hindered movement, and clumsiness in performing clinical tasks as reasons for noncompliance.

Obvious situations such as an artery surging out pints of blood are not the only danger. Maureen, an RN in another emergency service, arrived for a 3:00 P.M. shift, finding the usual backup in evaluations. First on the list was a man with vague complaints of intestinal discomfort. Basically he was fine, calmly sitting in a chair, his wife beside him. Maureen went to do his vital signs, figuring she should get a data base started on him. Simple enough stuff.

"Sir, can I have your arm to take your blood pressure?" she asked after introducing herself.

He extended his left arm. She wrapped the cuff around and put the stethoscope in place. It is her preferred method, as she was taught in school, to support the arm, to cup the elbow with her hand so that the patient isn't bearing the weight for those few minutes. It's a nice, reassuring thing to do.

She placed her hand gently around his elbow, pausing as she felt a scratchy ripple against her fingers.

"Excuse me," she said to him. "But what's under there?"

He moved his arm around so that she could see. The area was covered with fresh needle tracks with fresh blood clots all over them. Her fingertips had dislodged one, and a little sap was trickling down. He just kind of shrugged with a sheepish grin.

"An alarm went off in my head: *'IV drug user! IV drug user*, and you are touching his blood!' Christ, you have to glove-up just to take a blood pressure.

"There's nothing like it when you've touched something you know you're going to wish you hadn't touched. I stayed calm externally, but you can't imagine the anger and fear I felt. I wanted to jump and shout, 'You motherfucker, I'd better not get it from you!' There's this feeling like your fingers are the size of balloons and filled with open lesions.

"And there's damn little support out there in the medical community. It's like with rape cases—blame the victim. All they do is criticize us for 'poor technique.' I had a flash in my head: 'NURSE DIES—CDC SPOKESMAN CITES POOR TECHNIQUE! She had a tiny rash on the inner aspect of her left earlobe that left her vulnerable. . . .'

"Well, screw that."

Much of the apprehension is infused with anger about how those who do become infected are treated by the hospitals they have committed to. A frequently mentioned case is that of Hacib Aoun, a cardiology resident at Johns Hopkins who became infected in 1983. At the time, the twenty-seven-year-old Venezuelan had been caring for a teenage boy with leukemia who had been given several blood transfusions. Aoun had collected a blood sample in a glass tube that shattered as he prepared a blood test, driving a shard of contaminated glass into his finger.

In 1983, the human immunodeficiency virus (HIV) had yet to be identified, so when he became ill, Aoun thought it was only the flu. But symptoms persisted, and in 1986, after an HIV test had been developed, he was tested and proved positive. Blood saved from the dead teenager also tested positive. By that time, Aoun had married and had a baby girl.

Aoun disclosed his situation to his superiors, who promised to treat the information confidentially. However, a job he'd been promised in the cardiology department evaporated, and another, in a clinic, came with strings attached, including an insurance package that would be inadequate to treat his illness. When he refused this, the job offer was withdrawn. Colleagues began informing him that they'd heard rumors that he had contracted the infection sexually. Letters from the university hospital's lawyers intimated the same, even asking for a list of past sexual partners. (In another much-publicized case, Dr. Veronica Prego, infected by a needle stick, met a similar response from Kings County Hospital in Brooklyn.)

Aoun filed a $35 million lawsuit against Hopkins for slander and libel. In December 1987, the suit was settled out of court for an undisclosed amount. Aoun had been in the United States on a two-year physician training visa. In January 1988, the Immigration and Naturalization Service, adding insult to injury, denied his petition for permanent residency, which would enable him to enter experimental treatment at the National Institute of Health.

The U.S. Public Health Service estimates that by the end of 1992, there will be 365,000 diagnosed cases of AIDS and 263,000 deaths. Yet, one half of a national sample of hospitals surveyed in a UCLA study had no contingency policy to handle the possibility of employees becoming infected. There is ample skepticism about how compassionately hospitals would respond. Hepatitis B infections, the most comparable blood-borne virus, is generally employed as a gauge. Somewhere between

6,000 and 12,000 health workers become infected yearly with hepatitis B. Of this number, approximately 250 die. It has not been uncommon for hospitals to dispute an employee's assertion that he or she was infected on the job, resisting payment of the worker's compensation.

Many nurses and other health care workers resent being caught in the middle of the social and political problems associated with the AIDS epidemic. The Center for Disease Control has revised its definition of what actually constitutes AIDS three times in nine years, more in response to social pressure than to any change in the illness itself. Insurance companies have excluded people who have tested HIV-positive, thereby igniting bitter debate and legislation that prohibits health care workers from knowing the status of patients. While scores of health care workers have been infected by patients, it wasn't until the first patient became infected by a health care worker that a fire storm of concern was ignited in the press and Congress about the rights of anyone other than the infected person to know his or her HIV status. Some caustically refer to AIDS as "the Holy Disease," exempt from the normal protocols followed with other communicable diseases.

"God forbid we'd treat this disease like a disease. You'd think it was a sin to test for a communicable disease. There's so much hypocrisy: on the one hand we're supposed to be committed to preventive measures, but if you're pro-testing of all patients, people act like you're a Nazi or something. I've actually had a doctor ask me, 'What difference does it make if you know you have it if it can't be cured?' Well, for starters, I think it would be good for someone to know if they *have* it so that they can exercise the responsibility of not *spreading* it. But how do you have the option to practice socially responsible behavior in not spreading it unless you know you have it?

"Everywhere else in medicine, it's Holy Writ that knowledge is sacred. Even if you can't do anything with it at the time, you still gather as much information as you can, both to help individuals and to enact informed social policy. There's always the hope that you can do *some*thing with that information in the future. But with AIDS, we're constantly bowing to social and political pressures that are counterproductive.

"I personally take offense to being kept in the dark. If it's because people are afraid they'll be stigmatized by insurance companies, then go fight the insurance laws. God knows they need to have a harness put on them. I'm committed to helping those in need, but let me treat people with as much awareness of what I'm dealing with as I can have."

Double-glass pneumatic doors open from the ambulance bay into a reception area. Security guards meet all incoming ambulatory patients, directing them to sign a roster and then proceed to a waiting room where vending machines are available and a TV plays around the clock to ease the passing hours. An admissions clerk sits behind a bulletproof window, taking down insurance information and starting a chart.

Patients are called to the triage room over a PA system. It is an eight-by-ten-foot office with one door leading from the entry hallway and another into the treatment area. Working the triage room is called being "in the box." Another, smaller waiting area—for patients escorted by police or those already triaged and awaiting a room—is located just inside the treatment area.

The emergency department proper is laid out in a rectangle, two parallel hallways often cluttered with machinery—EKG machines, portable X-ray machines, a crash cart or two—soiled linen carts, and trash receptacles. Each hall is lined with treatment rooms for speciality cases (obstetrics, respiratory, two telemetry rooms, etc.), any of which can be appropriated as the need arises. In the rear, there is a large general treatment area partitioned into curtained cubicles. At the back of one hall is the X-ray suite. The entrance to the psychiatric crisis service is at the end of the other.

Up front, dead center, just across from the nurses' station is "the big room" used for immediate-access patients—cardiac arrests, traumas, almost anyone who arrives unconscious or spurting blood on the marble-tiled floors—with a lot of space for the swirl of activity that accompanies them. Children coming in are the worst. Babies brought in doll-like, slack limbed, their mothers crying and screaming, "He's not breathing! My baby's not breathing!" Babies who are dead. Babies who are dying, having already turned blue, and no one knowing how long they've been that way.

For Kathleen, the other "worst things" are the really traumatic injuries, limb amputations or major car accidents that leave people terribly bloodied. Once she had a lady come in, a trauma code. She was young, around Kathleen's age, and not breathing. First, they put an IV into her arm. The important thing in a trauma code is getting fluid replaced. While the other nurses struggled to get the rest of the clothing off, Kathleen kept saying, "Where's all this fluid coming from?" Still in the process of cutting off her clothing, they didn't realize that farther up her arm there was a huge hole.

"Here it was that all the IV fluid we were putting in her was just gushing right back out this hole. It didn't do her a damn bit of good. She died. It's always awful when it's somebody young."

Three or four such arrivals can throw an entire schedule into overdrive, disrupting not only the working of the ER but reverberating throughout the house as designated staff members race downstairs to assist. If the patient is sick or impaired enough to warrant admission to the OR, an ICU, or inpatient bed, the strain intensifies. More and more, unexpected admissions are becoming the norm in hospitals across the country. Since Reagan's tenure, emergency departments—the most expensive niche in the entire health care chain—have become the place where the majority of America's thirty-seven million uninsured citizens receive their basic health care. In 1988, over half the admissions to hospitals in the state of New York were unexpected.

Such arrivals are the most common time when the line between a physician's and a nurse's responsibilities blur. Procedures that nurses perform but are not supposed to—for which they are not insured or clinically cleared to perform but that everybody knows they perform—are manifold and change from institution to institution, as well as from unit to unit within institutions.

"It's funny, in university hospitals nurses do much more than we do. They're insured for it and are kind of amused that we don't do things like blood gases or femoral sticks."

The femoral artery is one of the largest in the body, running down the inner thigh from groin to knee. Drawing blood from it can be dangerous. Blood pressure is great and severe hemorrhage a possible consequence. Still, a femoral stick is a painful necessity when blood samples cannot be obtained from vessels of the upper extremities.

One must apply strong, steady pressure for several minutes in order to form a clot strong enough to prevent spurting. In many institutions, including the one where Kathleen works, it is policy that only specifically certified physicians can draw blood from this site. In common practice, however, many nurses do so if the physician is busy elsewhere.

If a patient arrives and is truly sick—for instance, in obvious hepatic encephalopathy (an enlarged liver), such as an end-stage liver from alcoholism, for which the doctor will need an ammonia level before he can decide what to do—and the doctor is busy intubating someone else—Kathleen will not stand idly by for an hour when she knows what bloods will be needed. She'll do that femoral stick and hope to God she applies enough constant pressure to the puncture site so that it doesn't bleed out. She'll do this, or other restricted tasks, if she believes she can do so safely. And assuming she trusts the physician on duty to back her up if something goes wrong.

For example, a young man in his twenties arrived via police van. He had been hit in the abdomen with a baseball bat. He was vomiting blood and balanced a pail on his lap, wiping his teeth and gums with tissues after each retching output. He rocked slightly on the edge of a gurney to soothe himself, his breath choppy and shallow. Occasionally he whimpered and choked tremulously, "Please don't let me die."

Kathleen has heard this often—cried, screamed, whispered.

"You'll be okay," she assured him.

She started an IV line, drew blood samples, and told him she needed some urine to test for blood.

"It hurts to pee. . . ."

"I know, we just need a little bit. . . . Just relax and let it come."

She hoped for enough to send for a UA and tox screen. He'd denied drugs, but she didn't believe him. She rarely believes anybody who denies drugs anymore. Mostly it's crack cocaine these days. A 1989 National Institute of Drug Abuse study reported that the incidence of cocaine-related emergency room arrivals rose fivefold in five years, the number of cocaine deaths doubling. Some shifts, almost every patient Kathleen sees has a crack-induced complaint: cardiac arrests in people in their twenties; suicide attempts from the crashing depressions; the casual violence that pervades the life-style.

Dealing with druggies can be taxing, an occasion when it's difficult to maintain a professional dispassion, particularly when children are involved. A woman recently arrived in a tearful panic, screaming about her two comatose children in the car. There ensued an hour of frantic activity, staff running and lugging the kids inside, stripping them and inspecting for wounds, starting IVs, drawing blood and cathing for urine samples while making numerous attempts to get information from the mother amid her histrionics—"My babies! My babies! I just came in and found them that way." She was finally coaxed into telling the truth. She'd given the kids tranquilizers.

"I thought it was just enough to put them to sleep. I just couldn't stand for my kids to see me using drugs" was her explanation. "You understand, don't ya?"

Kathleen wanted to grab her by her blouse and slap some sense into her.

Another kid, sixteen or so, high on crack and too many Bruce Lee movies, arrived with two broken legs, protruding ribs, fractured jaw, nose and clavicle as well as multiple lesser fractures, lacerations, and abrasions from an attempt to prove he could leap over the roof of an oncoming '87 Mazda.

Kathleen placed a sheet over the lap of the young man with the urinal. The physician was at the next bed, behind the curtain, suturing another patient's lacerations while discussing the assault victim with Kathleen.

"I guess we'll need to drop an NG tube," she surmised while jotting an initial assessment note about his level of consciousness and estimates of blood loss along with lung, heart, and bowel sounds. Inserting a nasogastric tube is specifically forbidden to nurses in the ER, though it is routinely carried out on the inpatient floors. The reasoning is that the condition of people in the ER is more obscure, their malady not yet diagnosed. More damage might be done.

"I'm gonna be about twenty more minutes with this," he exhaled, exasperated, behind the curtain. Kathleen was aware of the severity of that patient's injuries. She could hear the snipping of scissors, the ratchet chew of hemastats. "But we'll certainly need one to test for blood to find out if it's just vomiting from trauma or if there's intestinal bleeding."

"I'll do it," she offered, trusting the relationship they had developed. Both were jump-in-and-help-out kinds of people. Each had covered the other's ass on many shifts. "No sense making him wait and dragging this out longer than we need to. Might as well have some lab results back to look at by the time you can see him."

"Great." He sighed appreciatively. "That'll really speed things up."

"No problem."

Had he been someone she did not trust, even if he'd asked her to do the procedure, one she had performed hundreds of times, Kathleen would have said, "Oh, I'm sorry, but we're not insured to do that here."

Case in point: a patient arrived with smoke inhalation resulting in upper airway damage. He needed a STAT (immediate) application of moist, humidified air, commonly referred to as "cold steam." However, there were no cold steam setups in the ER. She called respiratory but was told they were involved in a code in CCU. More than one respiratory therapist should be available at any given time, so Kathleen voice-paged them, STAT. No answer.

In the meantime, she put regular O_2 on the patient.

When the doctor came in, he asked, "Where's the cold steam?"

She explained what was going on. She noticed a funny expression on his face but didn't pursue it, busy trying to get an IV in this man who was not only drunk, verbally abusive, and physically assaultive but also an old drug abuser with next to no veins left in his body. Pretty soon four nurses and two doctors were trying to get an IV going, without luck. After he was restrained, a femoral stick was done and some blood got drawn. Kathleen took the vials and walked them up the hall to the lab.

He was her patient, but there were six other people working on him. She'd already taken his vital signs and needed to pick up his chart, which she assumed the admissions clerk had made up, so that they could start documenting what was being done to this man. It seemed the sensible thing to drop his blood off on the way.

Eventually, the line was started, treatment proceeded, and the shift went on.

A week later, her nurse manager told Kathleen that this doctor, who was the chief of the service, reported that she had not applied cold steam to this man. He'd never said a word to Kathleen, and he was someone she had worked with many times. He brought it up in an argument with the HN about why he thought her nurses weren't competent.

"Like who?" she had demanded. "Give me specifics."

"So he pulled that story out of his brainpan—that I didn't put cold steam on this patient. He didn't mention any of the background details or that I'd run bloods to the lab, only that I'd left the side of my patient. I don't know how he thinks the blood gets there; those vials don't grow cute little legs and go jogging. The patient needed his carboxyhemoglobin done, and done immediately, to assess the severity of the inhalation. He didn't mention that there were six people swarming all over the patient. He said I didn't 'prioritize' what needed to be done, as if I didn't grasp the significance of the situation.

"I saw it all written up in my file later on along with the head nurse's evaluation, after talking to me about mitigating circumstances, and her judgment that I was competent. I never confronted him about it; I just didn't think it was worth it. But I never trusted him again. He knew the details of the situation and decided to ignore them to make his point. That's just evil and self-serving. I decided not to deal with him any more than I have to. I never give him any extra help.

"Needless to say, I don't drop any NG tubes for him."

After working awhile in the ER, Kathleen discovered that one of its benefits was the ability to regulate patient contacts more fluidly than was possible when working on med-surg floors or in the units, to move from person to person, being as close and interpersonal or remotely impersonal as desired.

Kathleen deals face-to-face with a lot of people, many of whom she can't stand, like the demanding, entitled ones unable to comprehend why she doesn't think their pain ("This is important, really, it's been hurting me for *six weeks!*") is as critical as the bleeder in the back or the code in progress; or the acting-out suicides ("Hey, honey, I ain't changing. I may cut my wrists, but I wouldn't be caught dead in that cheesy hospital gown"). On balance, there are patients for whom, for whatever reason, she feels immediate empathy and for whom she'll make extra time. And there are those from whom she gets little pleasures, like listening to people mangle the language telling her, "My uncle died of roaches in the liver" (cirrhosis of the liver) or who are taking "peanut butterball" (phenobarbital) for seizures.

"I've got this ache in my tentacles, and I'm coughing up fling."

It helps to have cohorts on the staff with whom she can defuse. It doesn't take long to enter the "us against them" mode with all the needy faces who come calling.

Sometimes, the bizarre, unpredictable cases help break up the day. Kathleen walked in on a male patient once to change his IV. He was someone she had not admitted. It was a quiet, unrushed Sunday. She was working a bridge shift, 11:00 A.M. to 11:30 P.M. His nurse, on the phone arranging his transfer to the OR, hurriedly scribbling on a chart, asked if she'd do her a quick favor and change his IV site.

Kathleen said, "Sure."

He lay on his side beneath a sheet that covered him to the neck, a bit squeamish, tense, and vexed, but in better shape than she anticipated for someone ready to be launched up to the OR. The IV site had infiltrated, the needle dislodged from the vein, spreading IV fluid into subcutaneous tissue, but not badly, having been caught early. A little swelling, some discomfort—she'd seen much worse. She was in a good mood with time to be a "good nurse" and attend to emotional and psychosocial needs. She started chatting with him, trying to lighten his mood.

She fiddled with the IV tubing, making simple, "What a gorgeous day out, huh? I guess summer'll be here soon" types of comments. He halfheartedly bantered back the usual replies. Then she asked, "So, what brought you into the hospital?"

He got real cool, real quick. His body grew rigid, face hardening. She figured, "Ooops!" and busied herself with tubing coils.

"I'm quite sure you know *why* I'm here," he snapped after a second, very hurt and defensive. "Certainly the story has gotten around to everyone."

"Sir," Kathleen dropped into that neutral tone taught to be therapeutic, nonjudgmental. "All I know is that your IV had to be changed. I'm working a swing shift today, and I've only been here for a couple minutes. If my question was too intrusive, then I apologize. . . . You don't have to answer any questions that make you uncomfortable."

Of course, she knew that as soon as she was clear of the room, she would beat a beeline to the nurses' station to check the chart for details. Instead, he apologized for his snappishness and opened up to her. Earlier that morning, he and his wife had been in bed making love when he had introduced the idea of anal sex. He'd been cajoling her to try it for some time. Her objection was that she was afraid it would be painful. Attempting to convince her otherwise, he'd lubricated the handle of a broom and was demonstrating on himself when he slipped and fell backward on it, ramming it into his rectum and perforating his bowel.

As excruciating as the pain was, worse still was the humiliation of being transferred to the hospital. When fire rescue responded, they refused to remove the broom; their policy is not to remove objects from wounds. That's the surgeon's job. What they did was saw the broomstick in half to make it more manageable in transport. He had to be carried out on the stretcher on his hands and knees, ass up in the air. Of course, when the sirens came screeching up to the house, everyone had come to look—neighbors, strolling churchgoers, Sunday joggers, and biking enthusiasts. His wife put a sheet over him, but as soon as the spring breeze blew, it was gone.

"Film at eleven, right?" he tried to joke, voice cracking, near tears. "Christ, this has been the worst day of my life."

"I guess it'll be pretty hard to convince her now, huh?"

"Shit, I'll be lucky if she doesn't *leave* me!"

* * *

In the ER, nurses have more leeway to put brakes on patients who are obnoxious and abusive, to call security and say, "I'm not dealing with this one till he cools out. Next!" In situations where time equals treatment, there is little room for diplomacy.

The patient, a black male, twenty-three, with AOB (alcohol on breath), arrived via police van in handcuffs. They put him on a gurney, cuffing one hand to the rails after he attempted to bolt out the door. He had been stabbed; Kathleen could see why. As she tried to get him undressed, he expressed his discontent forcefully.

"Get your fucking hands off me. . . . No fat white bitch is gonna take *my* clothes off. . . ."

He continued in this vein despite Kathleen's explanations of his need for treatment, and the admonitions of the two officers accompanying him ("Hey, brother, chill . . . She's only trying to help you out"). He was emphatic about what he would *not* allow: he wasn't wearing a gown, he wasn't getting any blood drawn, he wasn't letting anybody listen to his heart or lungs. As a matter of fact, every one of them could just go fuck themselves.

He interrupted his tirade only briefly, to put the moves on a cute young nurse's aide being oriented to bedside care. When Kathleen attempted to clasp his uncuffed arm in order to take his blood pressure, he jerked away, fisting his hand up to her face.

"C'mon, bitch, touch me, just touch me. . . . I'll shove that fucking thing right up your ass."

"Okay." She stepped back, rolling up the cuff, removing the stethoscope from her ears. (She shared a common fear that one day some belligerent or confused patient would clap his hands against it, rupturing her eardrums.) "Officers, you can take him out of here."

Of course, as soon as he was taken outside, he wanted back in. This cycle repeated itself three times. It took place in the big room, a diversion for the half dozen or so alcove patients awaiting their turns, shaking their heads, snorting disdainfully. One guy, with a tattoo of an owl or an eagle on his forearm, third on the list, cracked his knuckles and offered to slap the crap out of him if it would help speed things up.

"Finally, he became so foul and offensive that I lost my temper. This, nurses are never supposed to do. Anyway, when he started up the third time with the threats, I was standing there with the IV box in my hand, and I just told the cops, 'Okay, fine, he is out of here! He is not being treated in this ER at this time. . . .'

" 'And you,' I said directly to him, 'You can go to another hospital or back to the street to bleed. You'll be back in here unconscious, and we'll treat you then. . . .' (It has happened before that we've had patients who've been a pain in the ass, left, and were brought back unconscious so we could treat them.) 'But you get out of here right now. If you think I'm gonna stand here and be abused by you, mister, you're nuts!'

"So he was shouting as the cops took him out in cuffs, screaming about how he's gonna fuck me up. In this ER you hear a lot of that stuff: 'I'm gonna get you tonight in the parking lot, bitch!'

"I didn't know she was there, but the director of nursing was making rounds and overheard most of the exchange. She came up to me and said she supported my decision, which surprised me. It's all too common that people think they can talk to nurses any way they like—physicians, patients, family members. They can use the foulest language and you're never allowed to lose your cool. Hell, if you're *abrupt* with them, you hear about it."

Less than a decade ago, when Kathleen worked on a geriatric floor, it was not unusual for patients to remain hospitalized for a year; anniversary parties were held for them. She recalls one woman who waited nine months for placement in a nursing home.

That is unheard of today; two months is a long stay. Open hearts go home in ten days. It is the norm for patients to be discharged "quicker and sicker." This since diagnostic-related groups (DRGs) were introduced in 1983 as a means of curtailing rising health costs.

In the ER, DRGs translate into stricter criteria to gain entry into hospitals. More severe degrees of illness or impairment are required. It leaves Kathleen very uneasy. The anger engendered by DRGs pervades the system. Those who have worked both sides of the 1983 DRG division attest to increased tensions in hospitals. Patients and families are angry because they find themselves in a time of crisis without the amount of insurance coverage they believed they had, feeling abandoned and bewildered by vague regulations and restrictions.

Health care workers in general are angry because they feel hindered in giving the quality of care they entered their professions to give.

Physicians see DRGs as an intrusion on their professional autonomy and livelihood, lowering their standard of living, compelling them to see more patients. During the first seven years of the DRG era, the major impact was on Part A of Medicare reimbursement (the part that pays for hospital costs), while Part B (that covering the physician's bill) was generally unregulated. In many ways, this imbalance of vested interest between hospitals and physicians led to battles that were often acted out through the treatment of patients. As of 1990, though, Part B has started to become more regulated. For the first time, doctors are being held accountable for the quality of care they render to patients and are made to justify the time it takes them to do so.

Nurses are angry because, in the hospital's need to conserve costs, many workers who had been hired to perform ancillary tasks have been fired, and nurses have had to assume their tasks, tasks that nurses fought for years as a profession to be free of, tasks not requiring the degree of educational preparation demanded of RNs, tasks that take nurses away from administering the direct patient care they became nurses to perform. They are also angry because, as the person most accessible to patients, they are the recipients of patient anger and confusion about how it all works.

Ten years ago, if somebody came into an ER with blunt trauma to the head from bumping it on a car window—even if he didn't have a little knob or laceration—an X ray would have been done: "No fracture to the head. Still, he could have a concussion, so let's admit him overnight for observation."

Today, that same person can have the biggest knob on his head, requiring sutures, and be a bit lethargic, maybe feeling a bit goofy when he wanders in, and he will be sent home with a piece of paper for some significant other: *Wake every two hours tonight.* The instructions then proceed to describe a list of neurologic signs to check for. *If the patient starts to vomit or is unresponsive to waking or painful stimuli, initiate emergency transport to the nearest emergency room.*

"When patients yell at me, I just explain that, 'Yes, you're right, ten years ago you would have been admitted, but not today.'

" 'But, you don't understand,' they'll say. 'I've got the best insurance. I have Blue Cross and Blue Shield!'

" 'Well, ma'am, it has nothing to do with how good your insurance is or isn't. . . . It's because of how the government won't co-pay for certain things . . .' and on and on, trying to explain the new realities, the complexities of allowed and disallowed services and benefits, which seem to change from month to month and which I barely understand myself.

"A lot of times it gets reduced to a racial thing or a 'You call yourself a nurse? You say you're here to help people!' guilt-trip kind of thing—like I'm the one who devised the system—or a 'If it was your family member, I'm sure you'd feel different' kind of thing.

"You want to say, 'Believe me, I know how you feel. I sympathize.' But you can't. They don't hear it."

Doctors are in a better position to buffer themselves from such complaints. Kathleen has had ER physicians write discharge orders—"Inform patient of discharge"—that specifically shield the doctor from the patients and their bewildered rage.

"Discharged!" the patient then screams. "What the hell do you mean, discharged? You're not a doctor. I want to talk to the doctor. You don't know what you're talking about."

"The doctor wrote the order to discharge you."

"Well, lemme talk to him. I'm not leaving till I see the doctor."

Of course, the doctor refuses to walk the forty feet down the hall to inform the patient of his decision face-to-face. There have been times when security has had to be called to escort patients out.

> "Between the DRGs and the doctor's attitudes, sometimes you're just the brunt of a lot of anger. Not to mention the normal anger nurses are heir to because you're dealing with people who are at stress points in their lives. Or their relative is sick. You learn in nursing school that you'll have to deal with that, but then you get this other crap that you just don't need."

It is hoped that the person sent home has someone there to help him. Or that that person even has a home to go to. The cops brought a guy in to be evaluated after a fire in his apartment. Drunk, he'd fallen asleep in bed, smoking. His still-smoldering clothing was swiftly cut off so that he could be examined, but no burns, swelling, or other problems were found.

"Okay, he's discharged," the doctor told the nurse.

"What, ah, do you mean he's discharged?"

"Discharged, out of here, *his-to-ry* . . ." he sassed, his tone catching the attention of other staff members. He was a brassy pain-in-the-ass intern with a bad attitude, interdisciplinarily disliked. "Do I have to spell it for you?"

"Well, we're gonna have to wait a bit. . . ."

"No way! Get'm outta here. He can go—*now*!"

"But his home burned down. Where are we gonna send him?"

"I don't care *where* you're gonna send him. What'm I, the only one with a brain here? Just tell him to wait in the waiting room. Do I have to tell you everything?"

"But he has no legs, *doc-tor*!" she replied. The patient was a double AKA (above knee amputee). He had two stumps and no clothes, since they were discarded after being dunked in water. "Are you seriously suggesting I put a gown on this man, wheel him into the waiting room, and let him sit there?"

"Good question." A resident nodded.

"Inquiring minds want to know," Kathleen chimed in.

"He has no legs, no prostheses . . . ." the treating nurse continued, on a roll. "And he smells like smoke . . . I think that's gonna look *real* bad."

"First we had to find out if he had any place he could go. I mean, would a shelter take a man with no legs? They'd probably see it as a dump job for them and never help us out again. We spend a lot of time on the phone here, doing social worker, placement kinds of stuff. And, since DRGs, the resources just aren't there anymore.

"Of course, the patient was intoxicated beyond belief, so he couldn't tell us who to call or even if he was dead or alive. The only thing he could do was curse up a blue streak, just screaming at everyone.

"He had the kid in the next bed terrified of him.

"I tried to reassure the kid. 'He can't get to you,' I told him, lifting the sheet. 'See, he has no legs.'

" 'Yeah,' the kid said. 'But he's got *long arms*!'

"It helps to laugh. Sometimes it's all you can do."

5

"A Human Crisis"

Psychiatric Emergencies

Kenny Z., thirty-three, awoke Sunday morning with his Saturday suspicions intact. Lately, he'd been getting the threshold feeling that something was wrong in his household. His wife Brenda had been pestering him lately to cut back on his cocaine intake, even enlisting the aid of the kids in asking him to stop, using "but-Daddy-we-love-you" guilt tactics. She'd gone so far as to call the police last week after she'd practically forced him into bouncing her off the wall because she'd hidden his stash.

"I'm only trying to help you, baby," she'd insisted, trying to mollify him, but more likely she had another man and they were trying to steal his stash away from him.

There were lingering signs that something was amiss. He'd noticed lately how she had her dirty clothes piled on the floor in the corner, behind the chair. What was *that* all about? The chair itself was moved away from the wall, just a bit more than it used to be. That had meaning for Kenny, but nothing he could pinpoint. He'd confronted her about it in that argument the other night, but she just acted dumb, telling Kenny he was talking out of his head. That was before she'd called the police, and that young stud cop with the black leather gloves and the bench-press chest arrived, and she got all flirty and into that "thank-you-so-much, Officer" bullshit with him. She really must think he's a moron.

Something just wasn't adding up. Figuring that a few more tokes would help clarify things, Kenny had a quick hit from his pipe on the way to the bathroom, just enough to clear his thinking while he thought this all through.

Family sounds and kitchen smells rose up the stairs to meet him as he returned from the toilet. In the hallway, in mid-stride, his suspicions were confirmed. He was met by the Man Who Stepped Out Of The Wall. Right out of a crack in the Sheetrock! Kenny had to blink and refocus his eyes. They caught each other by surprise, freezing a moment in place, face-to-face, before the man dashed into the bedroom.

"Hold it right there, motherfucker!" Kenny shouted, racing in pursuit.

"Kenny?" He heard Brenda call him as he entered the bedroom, catching a glimpse of the man diving beneath a floorboard. There was a loose one, neatly hidden by the pile of Brenda's dirties, which explained a whole lot. Her lover had been hiding under the floorboards of his own bedroom! There was a part of Kenny Z.'s brain that wondered how this could all be possible. But this thought was less powerful than the swelling rage and justification he felt as he vaulted their bed and retrieved his revolver from his dresser drawer.

"I've got you now, you son of a bitch," he shouted. "You might as well come out of there. . . . *I said come out of there.*"

When his command was ignored, Kenny fired the first round a half foot to the left of the loose board. He heard his wife scream downstairs.

"Brenda," he called over his shoulder. "I've got your sweet man cornered, and I'll kill him if . . ."

She was wailing, "Oh, my dear God!" downstairs, and Kenny was distracted enough to catch only a peripheral glimpse of the floorboard man exit from a crack in the wall, take two good strides across the room, and dive amid the cushions on the couch near the window. It was a hand-me-down gift from his mother. He felt less in control of the floorboard man now, like he'd escaped Kenny's trap.

"Damn!" Kenny hissed, firing two rounds, bits of upholstery flying upward. He could catch no glimpse of the man in the holes he'd created. The floorboard man continued to ignore Kenny's commands to surrender, even when he promised not to harm him.

Brenda Z. scrambled out of the house with her startled children in tow, heart jackhammering, too terrified for tears. The first bullet had torn downward through the ceiling, spraying the room with dust and shattering the face of the wall clock five feet above her high-chaired infant's head. She didn't stop for the two blocks it took to reach a public phone that worked.

The police were useless.

"Ma'am, if we didn't see it happen, then there's nothing we can do about it."

"But there are bullet holes in the walls!" Brenda cried into the receiver. "It's a row house, for God's sake; he could shoot somebody next door. . . ."

"We haven't received any complaints from that vicinity."

"You mean you won't arrest him until he actually kills some . . . ?"

"Unless an officer witnesses it being done. . . ."

"Well, what'm I supposed to *do*?" she pleaded. "I have three small children with me. I can't go back there. Their father is shooting the house apart. That crack has him crazy. Is there *any*thing I can do? I'll do anything—swear out a warrant for attempted murder, what?"

"What you *could* do is to file psychiatric commitment papers that say he's a danger to himself or others. If you'll do that, then we can pick him up."

"Fine. Anything. Where do I go?"

"Go on over to the hospital and ask for the psychiatric emergency department. They'll tell you what you need to do."

The psychiatric crisis service (PCS) is the mental health equivalent of an emergency room. Such services were set up during the "deinstitutionalization" era of the sixties and seventies as a means of helping to keep the psychiatrically impaired population out of hospitals and functioning in their communities. It was meant as a more humane—as well as cost-effective—treatment alternative to lengthy incarceration in drab, impersonal state facilities. Good intentions, however, were easier to supply than dollars, and the entire system has been consistently underfunded.

This city is divided into "catchment areas," with designated outpatient clinics, inpatient units, and crisis services. The system is loosely overseen by the Office of Mental Health (OMH), located in city hall. OMH officers possess the power to issue warrants, commitment papers based on sworn eyewitness accounts, allowing the police to bring individuals into the crisis service—by force, if necessary—for up to five days of observation and treatment. It is rare that anyone remains in a crisis service that long. Assessed first by the nursing staff and then a psychiatrist, all are either admitted to an inpatient unit, where they'll await a hearing in five days, or are discharged within twenty-four hours.

The PCS in this hospital is small, tucked off in a corner behind the emergency department. It consists of a nurses' station, a couple of offices for conducting interviews, two seclusion rooms, and a bathroom with toilet, sink, and an often overflowing shower. There is also a "waiting room," two painted cinderblock walls lined with facing chairs with just enough room to walk double file between them. Seclusion rooms are a common feature in most psychiatric facilities. They are eight-by-ten spaces furnished with a mattress. They are used to lock away patients who are violent. If there is a danger the person may harm himself or others, he is restrained with leather cuffs and straps to cleats in the floor.

There are two gurneys in the hall, secured by braces in the wall, to which any overflow of violent patients can be restrained. The gurneys, seclusion rooms, and offices double as sleeping areas with foam mattresses the width of bicycle tires laid on the floor for nonviolent patients who need to spend the night.

The nurses' station is very cramped. It's difficult for two people to pass without weaving to make way for each other. On weekday shifts, when most staff are present—two psychiatrists, an RN or two, a social worker, and two intake workers—it becomes particularly congested. Everyone has less a work station than a shared circuit, each angling for a desktop to do paperwork. Because the crisis service actively intersects with the legal system, the charting is voluminous.

"Off shifts,"—evenings, nights, holidays, and weekends— are less crowded, and that suits Frank fine. Frank is the night shift RN, 11:30 P.M. until 8:00 A.M. Working with him are an intake worker ("sort of a pesudo social worker"; part of the nursing department and accountable to the nurse in charge) and a psychiatrist. Off-shift psychiatrists rotate through on an irregular basis, moonlighters from other hospitals. Usually they are fourth-year psychiatric residents picking up extra cash and rounding out their education in the fast and dirty world of emergency treatment.

Some residents are very good, able to make quick evaluations and treat aggressively. Sometimes, however, they are inexperienced and reluctant to make decisions. It's important not to become bogged down in prolonged periods of observation and evaluation, the hallmarks of traditional psychiatric treatment. "Treat'm and street'm" is the operative phrase. At times, the RN on duty must support and direct new psychiatrists, reorienting them to the realities of "street psych" as opposed to textbook interventions. In this, Frank has the secure backing of the supervising psychiatrist.

The crisis service is part of a citywide system. The primary objective of PCS is to remain "open," available to treat voluntary walk-ins and those like Kenny Z., who are brought in by the police against their will. There is an official cap of four patients at a time in the unit, though this is often exceeded. When the service backs up, going on divert status—because evaluations are being performed too slowly or no beds can be found for those being held—the entire system becomes clogged.

Frank's gravitation to psychiatric nursing began in the associate-degree program he attended in New York City. As part of his final semester, he took an elective clinical rotation in a crisis service in Spanish Harlem and worked with a nurse and psychiatric resident in a mobile unit that covered five emergency rooms. They did twenty to thirty consults each shift. Lots of drugs, lots of psychosis. He went along on several hostage calls.

One of the first involved an elderly man who had been held captive for several days by his psychotic son. Nobody could get into the apartment. The police declined jurisdiction, stating he was a mental patient. Frank accompanied the head nurse and psychiatrist to the apartment building, where they were met at the gate by the knife-wielding son. It took two hours to talk him down, convince him to surrender his knife and take some medication. He allowed them to enter the unheated, dimly lit apartment. The old man was dehydrated and very sick, an unmedicated, insulin-dependent diabetic. The son eventually permitted them to contact the rescue squad and transport his father to the hospital.

"It was very frightening, but fascinating. The head nurse and psychiatrist did a really fantastic job. You get that adrenaline rush, like in a code, and you do things you wouldn't do ordinarily. I was gung ho as a student. I was hooked."

Kenny Z. was immediately sequestered in seclusion and restraints when he arrived at PCS. Obviously stoked on coke, he belligerently screamed and cursed. He was accompanied by seven sweating police officers who had struggled mightily to get his wrists and ankles cuffed. One of them was the very same young stud, black-leather-glove cop with the bench-press chest Kenny had suspected as being overly solicitous with Brenda the week before. His presence only confirmed for Kenny that his wife meant to do him dirty.

"I want him!" he bellowed about the cop, demanding to be

left alone with him. "You get that pig in here, or I'll kick your ass."

In most psychiatric settings, restraints are a last-resort intervention, used only when someone has demonstrated that less restrictive options are not safe enough. In psych crisis, reverse rules apply: Anyone arriving with reported dangerous behavior is restrained straightaway, then released strap by cautious strap only when he or she has displayed adequate self-control.

Interviewing Kenny took upward of an hour. He was unable to speak below a shout, unable to sustain a coherent conversation without paranoid leaps of private logic and threats to anyone who hindered his will. He didn't deny his wife's allegations.

"If some son of a bitch was hiding in *your* sofa, what would *you* do?"

Upon admission, the staff pull together a coherent pattern of events by interviewing any combination of patient, family, friends, police. It's part of what Frank most enjoys, finding the picture in the puzzle, deciding if the patient requires hospitalization or can be glued together more speedily with medications and quick counseling. The majority of cases evaluated are involuntary arrivals, brought in by the police because commitment papers filed by family or friends state that their behavior is dangerous to themselves or others.

"Dangerousness" consists of overt attacks on others (chasing mom around the house with a baseball bat), self-mutilation (slicing oneself up with sharp objects, head banging, hand biting), or suicide attempts. Another criterion is a pattern of not being able to care for oneself. Things like drastic loss of weight (being poisoned is a common paranoid fear), not washing oneself, being unable to sleep, stomping around the house slamming doors, wandering the streets at night, leaving gas burners on unattended, or urinating and defecating in the wrong room are frequently cited behaviors.

Like emergency services everywhere since the advent of crack, PCS has become clogged with cocaine-related psychotic episodes, often swamping the resources of the service. Many days, every patient seen has some overlapping drug or alcohol problem complicating his or her mental illness, but crack is the hands-down statistical heavyweight. While government studies have shown an overall decrease in casual drug use in the last few years, there has been a significant surge in the numbers of people who are frequent crack users.

Staff members frequently wax nostalgic for the good old days of simple schizophrenia. The degree of psychotic behavior associated with crack use is staggering even to experienced staff members. Severe paranoia is ever-present, magical ideas of mind reading, thought insertion, and grandiosity commonplace, along with violent mood swings and zero impulse control.

Considerable energy goes into sorting out drug-related behaviors when commitment papers are filed, staff redirecting petitioners to detox-treatment settings. Forced treatment for addictions is not legal. But sometimes the violence is so compelling that staff members are willing to sidestep someone's rights temporarily in order to allow the family to make emergency arrangements.

The only thing that swayed the staff to file for Kenny Z.'s apprehension was his overt danger to his children. Otherwise his cocaine use would have been highlighted and the petition refused by the OMH. Brenda Z. was given the bad news bluntly: the longest Kenny was apt to be held would be twelve to twenty hours, depending upon how long he slept. She was encouraged to plan accordingly.

Kenny was given the usual "psychotropic cocktail" employed for such patients; 10 mg. of Haldol (a potent antipsychotic), 2 mg. of Cogentin (to avoid side effects from the Haldol), and 2 mg. Ativan (a minor tranquilizer, sort of a cousin to Valium). Because he refused to take the medication orally, injections were administered. Security guards and nursing staff held him down lest the needles break as he thrashed about, screaming, "Don't put that poison in my brain!" A towel was placed over his mouth as he spat and tried to bite.

Coupled with the "toddler car seat effect" of restraints, the medication had him asleep within an hour.

PCS has its own entrance. Those voluntarily seeking treatment come into a foyer where they are stopped by a single locked door, lead-framed with a sliding shatterproof, Plexiglas window. A lot of "token triage" is done at the door. Transit tokens are kept locked in the narcotics cabinet to be dispensed by the RN to all who can go elsewhere. Those with drug and alcohol problems are directed to detox centers. Those needing a place to sleep are sent on to shelters.

Everyone who rings the bell is supposed to be assessed before the door is unlocked and admission granted. Failure to do so can have serious consequences. Frank learned to demand to see everyone's hands before opening the door. He was once held captive in the doorway for a breathless half hour by a man toting a Molotov cocktail. The guy kept flicking his lighter ominously, threatening to ignite the gas-soaked towel hanging from the bottle's spout unless Frank convinced the hospital to allow him to visit his girlfriend, who was undergoing surgery.

"I just gotta tell her I'm sorry," he kept repeating tearily with alcohol-slurred speech, his mood oscillating between morose remorse and rage. "She's just got to know I'm sorry."

"Sure. Of course," Frank agreed in his most therapeutic voice, not knowing what the hell he was talking about, but encouraging him to supply more detail, talk it out. Frank kept wondering: if he slammed the door and bolted, could he make it around the corner before the explosion blew the door off its hinges and crushed his spine, or the fire engulfed him? He didn't think so, so he kept him talking until the 911 call placed by a security guard was answered.

Finally, two cops arrived. Flinging open the outermost door, they drew down on the man, shouting, "Don't make a move!" They scared Frank and the bomber, statue-stiff. Frank, surely in the line of fire, held his breath and tried to blend into the wall.

"Just put the bottle down slowly on the ground," one officer commanded.

The man looked at the bottle, then at the guns, and simply said, "Okay."

The scene made for a great bar room story. It's the kind of stuff psych staff savors.

Almost two thousand people were processed through PCS in the first six months of 1989. Patients are divided chiefly on legal rather than psychiatric grounds, whether voluntary or involuntary patients. Both groups share common symptoms. When drugs are not involved, the person is usually someone with a chronic mental illness who has ceased taking his or her medication. Soon the painful symptoms of psychosis start to recur—voices in the person's head cursing or commanding actions he doesn't wish to perform; paranoid delusions such as the TV or radio speaking about him, belittling him; inability to sleep; rapid mood swings; spending lavish amounts of money; confusion, nonspecific fears, and sometimes violence.

Voluntary patients are able to recognize the need for help or are willing to be swayed by family or friends into seeking treatment. The recidivism rate is high, and staff members become very familiar with many patients. Most are medicated, counseled about the need to continue outpatient treatment, probably throughout their lives, and sent back: to families or boarding homes, to community clinics or partial programs, to day-care centers or the nearest warm sidewalk vents. In the land of a thousand points of light, such "Band-Aid treatment" is often the best the system has to offer.

Frank tries not to dwell on what can't be done. He frames his thoughts about the system in terms of "the hospital's mission to the community." His anger becomes too intense when he considers a system where shortages are the norm: limited space and understaffing, an ineffective outpatient system—"the psychiatric archipelago"—where financial resources are ever-dwindling, treatment facilities disappearing, and the street population expanding. Often it seems that those requiring treatment are the only part of the system in a growth cycle.

The "boarding-home-dump-syndrome" is a common frustration: a patient who has been stabilized is discharged into the care of a boarding house proprietor who has no knowledge whatsoever of psychiatric-management technique. There is no structure—no group therapy, no support system, no expectations, no transportation to a clinic—and that person stops taking his medications, soon becoming a management problem. At that point, the patient either wanders out or is thrown out, but soon enough he is on the street again. Three months of hospitalization, medication stabilization, outpatient referral and placement—along with the massive financial investment those efforts represent—have been wasted.

Many people seen at the door are homeless, chronic street people, deinstitutionalized and disenfranchised. Some are unable to accept the treatment offered them, and there is no legal means to compel it. They have been kicked out by families or landlords who either cannot or do not want to deal with the bizarre behavior their illnesses provoke. They are evicted from apartments and homes, sometimes in the middle of the night. Many times they don't even have a psychotic process going on. Some just need a place to go to for directions.

Staff members hold differing attitudes about how much they should do in those cases. Once an abused woman showed up at Frank's door at three in the morning, a clear-cut "social car wreck" with five kids all needing a place to hide.

"You have a choice to make. You can do nothing for them, or you can try to help out. Some would say, 'It's not a psych emergency,' and without concern tell them that they have to go to such 'n such a place, a shelter or what have you, without finding out if they have money to get there, or if they have any medical problems.

"To me, that's not only a psych crisis, it's a human crisis. If a woman's out on the street at 3:00 A.M. with five kids and no place to go and no money, that's a pretty stressful event. Who cares how you label it? She's at risk. The kids are at risk.''

The freedom to make such decisions is what Frank finds most satisfying. As the only full-time RN on nights, he has had a great deal of influence in shaping unit policies. He is proud of the improvements he helped initiate since his arrival. Previously the service was often closed nights. Those seeking assistance were directed to call back in the morning. Today the service is active on a twenty-four-hour basis. Patients are processed and hospitalized, crisis evaluations are done along with family counseling and substance-abuse referrals.

Hospitalizing patients has become an increasingly arduous task during Frank's tenure in PCS. At first, DRGs had no impact on psych patients. In those innocent days, everyone believed it would be impossible to put a time limit on stabilizing mental illness. But within a few years, parameters crept into practice. Now when the team decides a patient needs admission, ''a tune-up,'' the shopping for a hospital bed commences. It is time to confront the insurance mix-'n-match monster. *If* the person has insurance, it's a matter of finding a hospital that will accept his particular type: if they have a bed available, if they are willing to deal with whatever behavior has been displayed, and if they will take someone with a particular diagnosis or a particular legal status on any particular day.

Then the insurance company has to be convinced that the person needs to be hospitalized, a post-DRG innovation. Outside of regular hours, insurance companies have numbers the staff calls to leave a message on a recorder. It may be hours or days before a return call is received. There have been instances where a call to obtain permission to admit someone to a five-day detox unit was placed on a Sunday and not returned until Tuesday.

The pace in the crisis service can change quickly. One moment no one is coming in, no phone or doorbell ringing. Sometimes it stays that way for hours. Staff members have played handball in the hallway to kill time. Then something somewhere sparks, and people start arriving back-to-back, ringing the bell, kicking the door. Needy, helpless, "gimme, gimme" people. Or police vans pull up, double-parking outside the door until it feels like a relentless parade of the forlorn and dysfunctional, the place emptying and refilling faster than a toilet tank.

"Then there's the Friday night melee when, say, during a code, a family gets into a brawl in the ER, trying to kill each other as their way of expressing grief. There's only a couple of security guards on duty. If we don't have our own fires to extinguish, we'll run out and jump into the fray. It's paybacks for all the times when security has pulled our ass out of the fire.

"It can get so damn crazy some nights. You feel like you're in the Alamo being overrun."

It's the unpredictability that Frank enjoys. An entire shift can tick off unnoticed while he hustles from evaluation to evaluation, chain-smoking, knee-length lab coat trailing over creased trousers and carefully polished shoes. The dress code is traditionally casual in psych settings. Almost any kind of street clothes is acceptable since uniforms are perceived as being intimidating to patients. Frank, however, is normally nattily attired with tie and nursing school tie tack, his only concession to comfort being sleeves rolled back to elbows, the "Don Johnson of dementia."

Political-turf battles abound between catchment agencies—patient "dumping" by police, "out of catch" referrals to jettison troublesome patients, refusals to take "diverts" when another service "closes." Each service believes that it pulls the lion's share of the city's load.

Frank keeps extensive records of anything that might be politically sensitive in the system or the community. Calling it "the

Frank File," he has gone so far as to photocopy documents to cover himself should a situation have the potential to blow up in his face. He learned this as a defensive measure when a physician in another hospital altered a chart after he and Frank became involved in a dispute. Having a photocopy of the original order sheet saved his job and possibly his license.

Systemic conflicts generally play themselves out with a lot of bitching, everybody writing up everybody else. Sometimes situations have developed tragically, even exploding into the news. In one instance, a patient dehydrated and died after waiting almost four hours in the back of a police van on a blistering August afternoon because every catchment service was backed up.

The worst police dump story at Frank's facility started with a 1:00 A.M. call from the police.

"Involuntary male. No drugs or alcohol, just crazy," the wagon officer said over the phone. "He's a wild one. Chased a neighbor with a butcher's knife. Says the neighbors have chipped in to have his head electronically wired. Their side of the story is that he's been eating out of their garbage cans, and they strung a trip wire to stop him. I'm just a lowly police officer; who's to say who's telling the truth? But my guess is he's one of yours."

"Sure sounds like it, but we're backed up. We're closed to involuntaries right now. We got a woman we're working up who sliced herself up pretty bad. She's kind of in and out of it, but my guess is she'll wind up in restraints. If so, that'll be in the hallway. We got a coke head screaming about killing Deborah Norville, and we just put another woman in restraints who tried to bite her left nipple off. Plus we have two walk-ins who have been waiting over an hour."

"Do you think you'll have room later?"

"Not before three-thirty. The nipple biter is scheduled to be transferred to an inpatient unit; that's why she's biting. The ambulance people swore to me they'd be here by three-fifteen."

"Well, what're we supposed to do? We have other calls coming in. We're the only wagon on tonight. We can't sit with this guy for over two hours.''

''Don't know what to tell you. Three-thirty's the best we can do. Sorry. Call OMH, I guess, see if they can send'm someplace else.''

''They don't have any place. They told us to call you.''

''Well, we can't take him now.''

''Well, *we* can't sit with him. I guess you're saying we have to let him go?''

''No, I'm not saying that. I can't tell you how to do your job. What I'm saying is that we can't handle him until at least three-thirty. What you do is up to you. . . .''

Seven hours later, an elderly woman awaiting a commuter train was grabbed in full view of horrified rush-hour onlookers by a man who flung her from the platform in front of an oncoming train. Forcibly subdued and detained, he later maintained she was one of the conspirators who had infiltrated his head.

· Conflicting stories circulated in the press. The woman's assailant had either been released from police custody or ''turned away from a mental health center.'' Recriminations rebounded for weeks, ''a thorough investigation'' promised.

Miraculously, the woman, devastatingly damaged, survived. Her attacker was returned to a state hospital, confirming the judgment of the inpatient staff who had treated him during multiple admissions that he was ''a man with headlines in his future.''

In the morning, Kenny Z. awoke, ruefully depressed, but clearer in thought, making the usual vows of abstinence. It's been said that sometimes the most you can hope for is having the patient go from saying ''Fuck you'' to ''Thank you.'' Kenny was fed and counseled about cocaine addiction, given referrals to voluntary treatment programs, and the locations and times of Cocaine Anonymous groups in his vicinity. He was given back all his personal possessions and discharged. It's known as the ''sleep, eat, and street treatment'' and is repeated every day.

Earlier, Brenda Z. had been called to let her know Kenny would be coming home. It is policy that when an involuntary patient is discharged, the petitioner is contacted—"informed" or "warned," depending upon one's point of view. The patient is given any referrals to outpatient clinics or support groups that might be helpful. Prescriptions are also given, if indicated. Free samples are routinely supplied to tide people over until they can be filled.

There are frequent disputes with family members when they are informed of a pending discharge.

"*What?* You're letting him go! You can't do that. Oh, dear Lord, no, no. What does he have to do, kill one of us?"

Frank tells them about having the locks changed.

"He breaks out the front window."

Frank tells them about obtaining a restraining order.

"I've had three of those. He doesn't obey them. And the cops won't come pick him up unless I file papers with you, and you tell me you can't hold him. Lord, this whole system is crazy."

Frank tells them about mental health consumer groups who are working to change existing laws, tells them about Al-Anon if alcohol is involved, Nar-Anon if there are drugs involved, tells them to complain to the district attorney, their councilman, the media.

"Ma'am, believe me, I know. I hear your frustration, and I sympathize. The system is lousy. We can agree on what *should* be, but we have to deal with what *is*. . . ."

There are lingering staff fears when certain patients are released. Not the majority by any measure, but some. Fears for the patient's safety. Fears for those they might harm. Fears they might have missed something. Fears for potential legal repercussions of the decision; there are currently three suits pending in this service alone.

Rose worked in a mental health center in Indiana that covered a six-county area. Technically, it was a thirty-six-bed inpatient unit. But because it was the only psych service available, nurses also did walk-in evaluations in the ER and phone contacts, "cold calls" on a crisis hotline, basic crisis interventions, triage, and referral.

The inpatient unit did little in the way of psychotherapy. Some behavior modification was used. ECT (electroconvulsive therapy, "shock treatments") was performed, more by some attending physicians than by others. Mostly patients came to have medication tune-ups. Turnover was rapid. Average length of stay dropped from fifteen to eleven days during the five years Rose was there. The unit was unlocked, except for four seclusion rooms. There were a lot of elopements, coming in spurts, requiring staff to chase people down the street and bring them back. Leather restraints were used when necessary.

It was a poor, rural area with a lot of people on welfare needing help. Nurses dispensed medications for indigent outpatients, administering frequent Pro-dec shots (Prolixin decanoate, a long-acting, injectable antipsychotic) and drawing blood work for Lithium levels, keeping the mania at bay. Drug manufacturing reps supplied them with plentiful samples. It wasn't exactly what Rose had envisioned when she decided to enter psychiatric nursing, but she was learning and expanding her repertoire of skills.

Rose chose to work in psych while in school. Her psych rotation was at a VA hospital during her last semester. Her instructor was very enthusiastic and inspiring. She wanted her students to have a good experience. There were eight students in the group. Like most of them, Rose was initially very uneasy with the patients. Many were Vietnam vets, young guys Rose's age who looked beautiful on the outside, but when they would open their mouths, such horrible stuff would come out. They would hide beneath the tables, shivering and rocking.

Rose was struck by the fact that she was able to help them feel calmer, more assured, coaxing them from beneath tables. That was very intriguing. At the end of the semester she felt much more comfortable with the work and thought she would like the challenge. She felt that with more exposure and knowledge, she could make an impact. It was also more comfortable for her than performing all the technical tasks required in medical areas. One of her teachers used to tell her she was very "chatty." It seemed the logical choice, combining the low tech with high talk.

Allison, a young woman from the undergraduate college, was brought into Rose's health center by her roommate in the middle of a night shift. Loud, legs rubbery, and dingy hair in disarray, she agreed to come only after threats of expulsion from school. Skunked on beers, she'd lost control, trashing her room and half the others along her dorm hall, doing a ferocious amount of damage before being intercepted.

She was demanding ("Can we pick up the pace here, people? I'm tired, I'm *really* tired. It's been a bad day. I've had enough of this reality shit to last a lifetime, if you know what I mean. . . . Now, how 'bout you just pick up the phone like a nice little nurse, and call the dorm madame and tell her I'm sorry, I'm *really* sorry—but, hey, shit happens, right? Anyway, let's get through here, and we can all get some sleep"); entitled ("These are the ground rules: You've got ten minutes to interview me—then I'm out of here. I'm sure these other people here won't mind if you just slip me in. I mean, *where* have they got to go?"); and affronted that a nurse would evaluate whether or not she would return to school. She was in therapy at the counseling center with a psychologist and expected Rose to contact him.

After the grandstanding and waiting her turn—"The door's unlocked, Allison, you can leave anytime"—she sat down with Rose for the formal intake evaluation, Rose jotting notes throughout.

Allison enjoyed an audience. Initially, her anger dominated: she'd ripped apart all her stuffed animals. She expressed vaguely homicidal ideations, wanting to kill this and that person who made her life miserable—her parents could be buried alive, which was how they made her feel; her teachers should be bored to death—but had no specific plans. She was negative for any psychotic features: oriented to time, place, and person; recent and remote memory intact; no delusional ideas surfacing, just some tangential connections, rambling self-referential speech, a tad grandiose. Most of it Rose attributed to the beer. Plus, she was barely out of adolescence.

The sluggishness of alcoholic remorse overtook Allison as they spoke, swathing her in a corrosive depression: she was "so lonely and empty," a yawning chasm opening around her life, especially at night; she was "such an idiot," how could she ever face the other students again? Christ, she felt excluded by the cliques on the floor to begin with—and now *this*. . . . She didn't have a boyfriend; got used occasionally for sex but didn't enjoy it. It was her birthday. Of course, no one remembered. No one understood her. . . . Or they saw through her and hated what they saw, just like she did sometimes when she looked inside. Her grades could be better.

When her apologies for yawning outnumbered her complaints, Rose judged her as being ready to go home.

Rose called the dorm supervisor at home, explaining why she didn't think Allison needed hospitalization. She informed her that Allison had agreed to go see her psychologist in the morning. Would the school feel safe taking her back if her roommate agreed to stay with her overnight?

It was acceptable, so she left.

Rose wrote it all up and moved on to her next patient.

Six weeks later, Rose was working day shift when another nurse burst into the medication teaching group she led. There had been a shooting at the college counseling center. A male counselor had been shot and possibly killed. It was on the radio. No details available. Rose was married at the time. Her husband, doing his master's thesis in social work, was employed at the center.

The phone lines were jammed. The police who knew didn't want to give a name out over the phone. It felt like forever waiting to hear he was safe. When he called, she cried. He'd been at a conference when it happened, but had learned some details. A female student had come in brandishing a handgun, saying she was going to kill her therapist. She was out of her head, crying and yelling and cursing. Another counselor, Larry, known to Rose and her husband—they'd been to parties together, gone out for Chinese food, the movies—stepped out of his office to see what the commotion was. She'd leveled and fired, hitting him square in the chest.

The gun's recoil knocked the girl backward unsteadily. Two secretaries pounced upon her, pummeling and kicking her, and grappling the gun clear of her grasp. Larry had been airlifted to the trauma center, but there was little hope he'd make it.

That afternoon, the word came down that the woman who killed the counselor was being brought into the psych unit for evaluation by order of the arraignment judge. She was to be confined to a seclusion room, since it was the closest thing to a jail.

"The judge thinks she's crazy," the sergeant in charge of the delivery detail confided to Rose, handing over a packet of paperwork and personal belongings. "You ask me, she's crazy like a fox."

Rose was one of the few people who didn't cluster to get a glimpse when the girl was brought in, loath to look at the person who'd murdered someone she knew, her stomach still turning. But it fell to her to do the admission note. She was still in shocked numbness, reading through the police report, wondering how she could speak to this person, much less evaluate her dispassionately, when she glanced at the attached ID photos, front and side view.

"Wait a minute." Rose read the name again, then returned to the photo, stunned. "I know this woman!"

She hurried to the seclusion room, overseen by two police officers. Winding a strand of hair around her index finger over and over, rolling it out, winding it back, Allison sat on the mattress and stared at her shoe.

"Allison?"

She looked up slowly, focusing on Rose without expression.

"Allison," Allison said as if considering the possibility, then nodded. "Okay."

Unit policy included keeping all outpatient contact sheets. Rose ripped through the files, going back six months. She knew it hadn't been that long. It was like her heart had stopped and her stomach was heaving, doing flips. She was plagued with guilty recriminations: Had she missed something?

Finding the sheet, Rose read it over and over, reinterpreting statements, observations, scanning for clues. She had other staff nurses read it, her head nurse, the psychiatrist in charge, the investigating officers. It became a piece of "evidence." There were insinuations of legal repercussions. It became the weightiest two-page document in her life since she'd memorized the Ten Commandments in parochial school. Upon close scrutiny, though, her documentation proved adequate. Everyone agreed there was nothing unusual about it, nothing they all didn't hear from dozens of drunks or kids in search of selfhood every month. Nothing that would lead anyone to believe Allison was capable of such an act.

"It's one of those things you just never know. It haunted me for a long, long time. I felt very bad. It still comes into my thoughts.

"I ended up working with her while she was evaluated as she awaited her court date. She stayed in seclusion for three months—not because of any bizarre behavior, but the fact that that was the only place we could be sure she couldn't elope from. I tended to keep her at arm's length. I dealt with my guilt, I think, by being angry with the charge nurse on the unit who spent what I thought was an inordinate amount of time with this patient. I felt she got overly involved with her.

"They wound up calling it a borderline episode [Borderline Personality Disorder, a type of character disorder with frequent lapses in self-control, self-mutilating behavior, and brief psychotic breaks], and she was eventually shipped out to a university psych research unit, where she stayed for about a year. When they wanted to discharge her, the family of the person who'd been killed was quite upset. There were more depositions and legal battles. It was dragged up in the news again. It was all very painful.

"You just never know. You try to learn as much as you can, to do the best job you can. But you just never know."

6

"That Long Hallway"

Medical-Surgical Floors

Kathy likes to arrive early for shift change so she can have a cup of tea in her hand when she sits down to receive report. These are often the only unhurried minutes she will have before bedtime. When working the day shift, she has to rise in time to get her kids ready for school before driving into the city. On those blissful days when she gets home earlier than the children, she can catch some sleep, a "nursing nap," before preparing dinner and helping with homework. Usually, though, the day runs straight through.

Each shift follows a series of ritualized procedures, beginning with nursing report. Some hospitals use "walking report," with oncoming and off-going nurses going from bed to bed, passing information with the patient present, each able to assess what has been accomplished and what still needs to be done. In other hospitals, report is transmitted by tape recorder or, most commonly, seated face-to-face. Kathy's floor uses this last method, usually in a conference room next to the head nurse's office.

Officially, the function of report is to convey all pertinent information about the patients each nurse will be responsible for on the shift. It is usually organized by bed number and includes the patient's name, age, race, diagnosis, and symptoms prompting admission, doctor, current length of stay (LOS), and the progress the patient has made toward discharge. Most of this information is noted within the tiny blocks of a Kardex. A Kardex is a clipboard-sized binder with index cards inserted into clear plastic sleeves, one per patient. Each card is specially printed with spaces for medication or treatment record keeping. It is possible to review someone's medication for up to a month at a glance. Nurses giving report commonly flip through the Kardex as a reference, conveying the most recent additions.

Unofficially, report functions as a time for socializing between shifts or as a chance to talk to a supportive listener about problems with patients, staff members, or administrators.

Before the previous shift's nurse departs, a narcotic count is done. Narcs are counted by both the oncoming and off-going RNs, each signing a pharmacy inventory sheet verifying that the number on hand is correct.

Because report is given by room and bed numbers—and not by the degree of patient illness and care required—Kathy immediately sets about prioritizing those things that need to be accomplished on her shift. The patient population reflects a variety of illnesses—hypertension, diabetes, congestive heart failure, pulmonary, gastrointestinal, and cardiovascular disorders.

Kathy usually starts off with those things that weren't done on the previous shift—return phone calls, check lab results, flag odd medication regimes, make sure this test is ordered, that X ray read. There is a well-known phrase in the field: "Nursing is a twenty-four-hour profession," meaning each nurse gets done what she can and passes the rest on to her relief. However, leaving tasks unfinished is very much frowned upon.

It's easy for Kathy to understand how things get overlooked or bumped from another RN's priority list. The interruptions are endless; if you don't keep track, bad stuff can happen. Once she had a tourniquet on a man's arm, about to insert a needle to draw blood, when a voice in the hallway yelled, "Help! Quick, help!" She dashed out of the room to deal with the crisis, someone hanging half out of bed, tangled in a loose Posey restraint.

Several minutes later, sauntering by the first room, she was hailed by that patient.

"Ah, y'know," he said apologetically. "My arm's starting to lose feeling."

"Yeah? Why's that?"

He lifted the sleeve of his hospital gown, and her jaw dropped. The tourniquet was still in place, biting into his fleshy upper arm, purply discoloration spreading.

There are a lot of near misses.

Kathy tries to keep on top of things by jotting it all down on a sheet of paper she calls her "brains." The paper has square blocks on it, each block representing a bed, where she makes notations—IVs that need to be changed, heparin locks that need to be flushed for a KVO (keep vein open) line, sterile dressings done and the times for each, *need to do now* items, those in the next hour and the hour after that. She carries this reminder sheet with her at all times, adding and deleting as needed. God forbid she would ever lose her "brains" when it comes time to chart at the end of a shift. It has happened, and she has been panic-stricken: "I don't remember half of what I did all day!" It feels like the end of the world.

Kathy makes a quick rotation to each patient room, taking vital signs and performing a head-to-toe assessment at the outset of each shift. This often leads to re-prioritizing her "brains"— maybe somebody has soiled themselves or an IV has become dislodged. A patient's condition can change in any number of ways since last being seen. When doing her rounds, she asks all patients to tell her what they need and adds the request to her "brains," her "whatever for whoever list."

"You might not see me for another hour," she always informs them. "But I'll get it for you."

Each floor is a block long, consisting of two parallel hallways, each the mirror image of the other. Patient rooms line the outer perimeter, allowing those rooms a window overlooking busy city streets. There are also patient rooms in the center, at the far ends of the hall.

The nurses' station is dead center, able to monitor elevator banks and waiting rooms. A utility room sits on either side of the nurses' station, one for each double wing. These rooms have treatment supplies, countertops for charting, and space often appropriated for quick conferences. Management-wise, the floor is divided into four sectors, twenty beds apiece, each covered by a "team" consisting minimally of two RNs, and an LPN or a nursing assistant.

Kathy's next series of tasks center around administering medications, beginning with "chart checks," an often awesome undertaking. Just finding a chart can be a challenge. Charts are housed in carousel racks at the nurses' station but are commonly appropriated to conference rooms, offices, hallways, or whatever niche can be found by someone who needs to collect his or her thoughts before scribbling a quick notation. Multiple disciplines require access to patient charts each shift. Nursing, medicine, social work, nutrition, physical therapy, etc.—each is responsible for ongoing documentation. And whenever someone wants a chart, he or she wants it *now*. Documentation is commonly the final act in patient contact. It's like a passport that requires stamping before one can move on to the next case.

Nursing chart checks consist of verifying all medication orders written by physicians for all patients against their transcription to the medication Kardex, which becomes a part of the legal document of the chart. This is usually performed by a unit clerk. If no unit clerk is present, it becomes the nurse's job. Nurses use the Kardex to document distribution of all medications, from aspirin and vitamins to narcotics, dating and initialing each dose. Nurses are legally responsible for seeing that medication orders are dated correctly (both starting and ending dates), that all orders are signed by a physician and correctly reflect the patient's condition, including the proper route, dosage, and frequency. If any aspect of any order is incorrect, it is incumbent upon the nurse to track down the physician to correct it before the medication can be administered.

The next steps in the medication sequence are pouring and dispensing medication. This includes pills and solutions by mouth, eye, ear, or nose drops, intramuscular injections, and

IV solutions. Medications are to be dispensed in "a timely manner." Most hospitals have set med schedules—9:00 A.M., 1:00, 5:00, and 9:00 P.M.—but it is rare the schedule is met. Interruptions throw things off throughout the day—emergencies, both minor and major, patients off the floor for treatments, etc. Plus there are many "off-time" meds to be distributed, depending upon a particular patient's problems.

If Kathy is covering ten patients, each may be on from three to fifteen drugs requiring administration from one to eight times per shift. She is responsible for knowing the main actions and potential side effects of each medication she administers. It is often two hours into her shift before she starts making medication and treatment rounds, pushing the medication cart room-to-room down the hall.

The cart is a block of plastic, chrome, and steel sitting atop four wheels. Standing about four feet high, it has been described as a flat-topped R2D2 with drawers. Each patient has a plastic drawer. A locked metal drawer at the bottom holds the narcotics. Some nurses carry the narc keys around their necks on a long cord. Kathy prefers to keep them in her pocket, having heard stories about being strangled by crazed patients.

Coming down the hall, Kathy has her cart piled high with all the things she jotted down on her assessment rounds—tape to retape the IV in Rm. 67 . . . a K-pad in Rm. 69 . . . an ace bandage to Rm. 71-A . . . footboard for the comatose patient in Rm. 71-B to avoid muscle atrophy . . . toilet paper here . . . ice there. The cart also carries standard therapeutic supplies— plastic sleeves filled with medication soufflé cups, packaged drainage bags, blood-sugar monitoring devices and urine dip sticks for diabetic patients, several packs of sterile pads and gloves, masks, protective eyeglasses, and multiple disposable packets of Betadine, the topical antiseptic solution of choice for wound care.

Kathy has a few personal items also—paperback quick reference guides for medication and therapy information, as well as a tube of hand cream for application after the dozens of times she washes her hands daily. She keeps these locked in the narcotics box, lest they disappear.

In med-surg nursing, especially, one has to constantly juggle a basket load of information. Any single bit of it might be trivial, but the collective weight often feels like a burden, each eating away the minutes in the hours of her day. Shortcuts are avidly sought in an attempt to lengthen direct-patient-care time—pour several consecutive med dispensations back-to-back while the drawers are open and pray new orders aren't written before they are given out; buddy up with another nurse to do patient turning rounds. Sometimes shortcuts lead to trouble or potential trouble. A year ago, a new policy circulated in Kathy's hospital: nurses' notes were placed on bedside clipboards along with vital signs and intake and output (I&O) flow sheets. The idea was to make it more convenient to write anecdotal notes at the time procedures were performed or incidents occurred rather than having to traipse off to locate the chart, scribble a note on a brains sheet, or try to recall it at the end of shift.

Because the pages remained at the bedside until filled, visitors had access to browse through them.

Kathy got into the habit of writing out a note of all the care to be delivered at the onset of each shift—patient turned at nine-thirty, noon, and two-thirty, meds given, IVs changed—when she did her initial head-to-toe assessment. It was a way of organizing her shift. She felt that if it were written, then she *had* to do it. That was her agenda. It made the initial rounds longer, but she felt it paid off in procedural tempo.

A relative of one patient read her notes and saw they were signed off for midnight. He was a tall black man, stuffy and self-righteous. He summoned her into the room several times during his visit, pointing out shortcomings in the care of his aunt. He was one of those people who, when a nurse disputes an opinion or observation, attempts to chastise her by saying, ''I guess we'll have to see what the doctor says about that,'' like that's supposed to leave Kathy quaking in her Dr. Scholl's.

When he called her in the final time, he had the clipboard in his hand. He held the board up to her face.

"Can you tell me, miss, what's the meaning of *this*?"

She scanned the last note where his index finger tapped.

"I don't understand what your question is," she finally said.

"*Why* are they written?"

"Oh, I often do that—writing out my paperwork when I have a moment." She shrugged. "I find it speeds things up with giving the care."

"Why, because she had a stroke and can't complain if you don't turn her?"

Kathy stared, dumbstruck. It finally dawned on her that he suspected she had been pre-charting to avoid the work. It was an interpretation that had never occurred to her.

"Sir," she said forcefully. "I have beliefs that say, 'If you write it, then you're duty bound to do it.' To me, that's like written in blood."

He observed her thoughtfully. She realized he was evaluating whether or not she was telling the truth.

"All right," he said gently. "I'm sorry if I offended you."

"Luckily, he believed me. I guess he thought it was too incredible not to believe. Otherwise, he could have hauled me down to the nursing supervisor's office, and I could've been in big trouble. Clearly, I stopped that practice."

Her worst assignment is having the last eight patients at the end of the hall. It's not because of the walking. It's because in order to get there, she has to pass the other rooms. Patients constantly cry out and call lights ignite over doors whenever they see a blur of white. It's worse still during visiting hours, when family members skulk by the door, beckoning as she passes, even though she has already explained that their relative is not her assigned patient.

Kathy finds it hard to refuse to help, knowing it's *always* an emergency when a relative is hospitalized. Usually it turns out to be no more than a bedpan scene, but the person always pleads, "Oh, no, please don't go. I'll be through quickly, I promise." So she stands there while the shift ticks away, knowing her own patients are waiting.

Of course, the bed sheets and blue pad always get soiled, so she winds up changing the pad and washing her hands, again. During this time that she is doing things that have nothing to do with her anyway, the family member is asking questions about things she has no information about. She tries to explain how to get the information they want, sometimes suggesting they ask a doctor directly. But patients want nurses to be conduits to physicians, not wanting to be perceived as "a bad patient."

Maureen, an RN in the same hospital, has experienced this often. Usually it's about things she has little control over, like a type of medication the patient may not like.

"Did you tell your doctor that?" she'll ask. "Did you *happen* to mention that to him when he was just in here?"

"Oh, no, I don't want to bother him. He seems so busy."

"Well, I'll certainly make a note of your complaint in the chart. I wouldn't mind passing this along to him, but I may not even see him. And I think he would hear it better if it were coming from you."

She has learned that nine times out of ten, when she passes such information along to a doctor, his response is something like, "Gee, I was just in there talking to her, and she didn't say anything to *me*." She is left being looked at like she's having a psychotic break and imagining the whole thing. She has even been asked, "Maureen, do you think the patient *should* want that? Is it *you* who doesn't like the meds the patient is on?" Physicians never seem to ask themselves, "What is it about me or my role that makes this patient fearful of approaching me?"

Kathy always tries to encourage direct patient questioning of physicians also.

"Couldn't you just ask for us, dear?"

"As I said before," Kathy states, "your mother isn't my patient. But I'll send her nurse down to talk to you if I see her."

"Thank you, dear. You've been so nice."

"What you learn is that when you've helped someone like that, the patient and family member feel like they've actually made contact with another human being who has responded to them. They decide they like you. So they'll call for you constantly."

Once Kathy is extricated, there are four more rooms to pass, each brewing a crisis, a gauntlet of guilt—somebody hanging halfway out of bed gagging, a family member arguing with a bypass patient but drowned out by the roommate, who's screaming, "Shut up! You're too loud!," an eighteen-year-old across the hall smoking pot under the covers with the door closed, his next-door neighbor bellowing, "Nurse, nurse, come quick—the football game is on and my television is broken! This is crucial. Call for help!"

Kathy has heard those stories about spontaneous combustion. Sometimes she prays it would happen to her.

In order to remain sensitized to how dehumanizing being a patient can be, Kathy sometimes recalls her experience during the birth of her second child. She was being prepped for a C-section and a spinal was being performed when her gown fell down, exposing her breasts. She couldn't move an inch, a needle stuck in her spine, when, as though on cue, a stream of ten strangers came strolling into the OR suite looking like a kindergarten line. Seeing this mostly male group in their short white jackets, she thought, "Oh, God, not medical students!"

As they wandered over to watch, not one person said, "Ah, Kathleen, do you mind if they observe?"

"Of course, I had my delivery on the day the oldest member of the medical group was covering. He's as antiquated and thick as lumber.

"I said, 'Ah, excuse me, but who *are* these people?'

"He ignored me. I asked twice more before turning to the nurse, another woman, who said, 'Oh, well, they're just going to witness the procedure.' She said it as if my body was somehow removed from 'the procedure,' but at least she was a little embarrassed. She knew what I was getting at, like: 'Did they pay to get in here?' or 'It would've been nice to have maybe mentioned that there were gonna be twenty extra eyes in here.'

"Forget about the woman anyway; it's as if when a woman goes into labor, she loses her humanity. So, they lay me down while they're all standing there, saying to me, 'Now just relax.'

"Relax, right!"

Kathy's favorite staff position was as an IV nurse. There was a lot of mobility. She roamed the house, a beeper on her belt. It was very social, dealing with a multitude of people—nurses, doctors, patients, and their families. If someone got on her nerves for two minutes, she knew she could be out of there quickly.

When I'm on the floors, Kathy had told herself in nursing school, I'm gonna do what I need to do as far as tasks go. Then, after I get them settled down with their back rubs, I'll be able to sit by their side and let some little old man tell me his sad story or let some young teenager tell me his fears or hold the hand of some dying person . . .

The reality turned out to be that when people were dying and they got a look in their eyes that asked her to linger longer—when she knew it was ten-thirty and she hadn't finished giving out ten-o'clock meds, and hadn't finished charting, and hadn't organized report for the next shift, who would be sauntering in by eleven o'clock—it was all she could do to keep from saying, "Yo, buddy, I know you're dying . . . but, hey, I don't have the *time*."

She wound up feeling miserable at the end of the shift, lapsing into the second-person pejorative on her drive home: Jesus, Kathy, you don't even have five minutes for a dying person?

But she didn't. And nobody else did either.

In IV therapy, though, she could be that role-model nurse, the person who could take the time. After finishing dispensing the pain part of it, if all went well with her techniques, she had the time to talk with someone about his or her concerns.

Every fifth week, she did chemotherapy. It often required spending an hour in the room, starting the IV, infusing the solution slowly, assessing the patient's ability to handle it.

Kathy found it to be one of her most rewarding experiences. Most people were terrified of the purposeful poison dripped into their veins. They were grateful for someone who wasn't clinically detached, someone who could sit and talk with them or simply look into their eyes with nothing to do but *be* with them. Some of her most spiritual moments in nursing occurred in such situations—sensing the bond that transcends social, cultural, racial, political, and economic barriers; allowing patients to become people.

Kathy was involved in an incident that grew beyond all proportion. On a Tuesday morning, a call came to her home from the head nurse of the floor to which she had been pulled over the weekend.

"It's urgent that I speak to her right away," she told Kathy's husband, who called her out of the shower.

Kathy took the receiver in one hand, toweling her hair with the other.

"I'm sorry to bother you at home," the HN, whom Kathy barely knew, said formally, "but I have to inform you that you're being reported. We had a patient here, one of yours, who had a pneumothorax [air or gas in the pleural cavity, a potentially lethal condition] Sunday. He had bad CHF, and you didn't call the doctor and get X rays."

"Whoa, let's put the brakes on a second," Kathy interjected, taken aback. "Can we take this from the top? Like, for starters, who's the patient?"

The HN named him and proceeded to relate a distorted series of events implicating her in poor management of a patient. Kathy's anger expanded with each accusation.

"Hold on a second," Kathy interrupted. "I think I'd better take notes so I don't miss these details." Shaking with rage, she went to get a pad and pen.

The incident had occurred on her Sunday shift. The patient was an elderly male whose condition began to worsen just after the onset of the shift—fever spiked, loaded lungs, respiratory distress.

She phoned the intern on call at 8:00 A.M.

"Oh, he's been like that" was his disinterested response.

"Well, this is the first time I've seen him," Kathy said. "When I got report, nobody said anything about this." The man was getting CVP (central venous pressure) readings. She'd been told to monitor him, yes, but nobody said that he currently—or even in the last few days—had been having a problem. "My initial assessment is that he's in bad shape. Since they didn't tell me about his trouble breathing in report, I can only assume that, a) they gave me a very bad report, which I doubt, or, b) that his condition has deteriorated."

"I saw him last night."

It was obvious he didn't want to be bothered.

"Yeah, but it's twelve hours later."

"Well, monitor his CVP."

It was high, about twenty, which Kathy considered abnormally elevated. The normal CVP range is between five and ten cm. A higher number indicates an overloaded fluid volume. She called the intern back at 10:00 A.M. because the man was getting worse. She begged him to come down and evaluate this guy.

"Listen, I can't respond to the whim of every floor nurse that calls me. I can't even fill all my own whims."

"Look, I realize you might be busy, but you could have one

of the other guys come down here for you. You have other guys
who work here on the same service."

"I don't ask other people to do *my* work."

"Well, I want you to know, I'm documenting that I asked you
to come down and see this man."

"Hey, do whatever you want."

At noon she called again. The intern finally decided it was
time to get a STAT chest X ray, telling her over the phone,
"When you get the results, call me so I can go look at it."

"Doctor, we're busy here, too. You know you've been called
three times. I'm telling you the guy's in bad shape. I'm sure you
can tell that I'm upset. You should know you've got to check an
X ray, okay?"

"I want you to take a verbal order—'STAT X ray and call me
with the results.' "

She wrote the STAT X ray part, omitting the rest, fetched the
STAT portable, kept in a closet two units away, and notified the
X-ray tech. Seeing him with the machine outside the room,
Kathy asked, "Did you get it done?"

"We've done two already."

"Two?"

"Yeah, we did one last night and one yesterday afternoon."

"I'm talking about the one you have to do *now*. Did you get
it or not?"

"Oh, ah, well, okay, I'll do another one, I guess."

By then it was 2:00 P.M.

Going off duty that day at four o'clock, Kathy told the others
in report about the X ray, that the doctor needed to evaluate it
and needs prodding to do so, that the patient is a real cliff sitter
requiring a close eye be kept on him. She then left.

Sitting on the edge of her bed, Kathy scribbled and listened
without interruption as the head nurse ticked off a litany of her
failings and the intern's interventions to assist the patient.

"When chief-of-staff rounds were done on Monday morning," the HN scolded, "the patient was in *severe* congestive
heart failure."

"Well, my God, what a surprise." Kathy sighed. "I've only had it documented since 8:00 A.M. Sunday morning—how the patient was in distress, how I'd called the doctor with CVP readings, vital signs, etc. How nobody came to see him. . . . But, all of a sudden, on Monday, with the chief of staff—who I guess was reaming out the doctor—it becomes a big deal, huh? All of a sudden it's, 'I told that nurse to call me when the X ray was ready. She didn't call me.' "

"Well, *did* you call him?" she asked, focusing only on that part of it, what the doctor said. It fried Kathy, one nurse not supporting another nurse, holding the company line.

"Well, frankly, no, I didn't. And it's not like it was out of malice or to get him in trouble, but because I was as busy with my own work as he is with his. Is there some reason to believe that a doctor is busier than I am? I had a code and two admissions that day. . . .

"And what about the two nurses who had that patient for the next sixteen hours? Did *they* call the doctor? I don't see where that should all fall on me. What, did the patient get *better* for those sixteen hours and then regress again?"

"Kathy, I want you to come in and talk to the chief of staff and the other doctor, the intern who was on call. And I want you to sign an incident report accepting responsibility for this."

Kathy was silent a moment, smoldering.

"I *refuse* to come in for that," she hissed, equally enraged and flabbergasted. "I refuse to accept accountability for a doctor's lack of interest in his patient. Did you read my nurse's note?"

"Well, no," the head nurse stammered. "Not yet."

"Well, I want you to read them from the time I came on. You'll see that I pursued him for coverage, and he either forgot or just didn't care about what he was supposed to do."

"But *he* said you were supposed to call him. . . ."

"Is that written anywhere?"

"No, but he told me he told you . . ."

"Well, then it's his word against mine, isn't it? I got the

X ray, as ordered. He knew the results would be up. I warned this man. And now you want me to sign something that will imply that *I'm* somehow deficient? I refuse, and you can write that I refuse! I stand by my notes. If you read them, you'll see that I'm covered.

"I cared about that patient. His vital signs were written for twice a shift—even with a CVP line in!—and I took them every half hour to an hour. I treated him like he was in a mini-ICU. With *no* support, not a shred of help. I was there with one other nurse and one aide for twenty-eight patients. I even called the supervisor and told her that the doctor wasn't responding. She said, 'Well, I'll see if I can find him. . . .' Nothing happened. I documented that, too.

"If you read my notes and find you're not satisfied with my performance, then maybe it's time for me to leave the hospital, but I absolutely refuse to take the flak for him for not following up!"

She was breathless, trembling. It was the first time in her life she ever did anything like that, as far as refusing the request of an authority figure. It was cleansing.

"Well, he's here. . . . Would you like to talk to him?"

"For what—so I can argue with him? He's mad because he's in trouble with his top doc. And he *should* be in trouble! He knows what he should've done. I'm not his personal secretary who exists to remind him of his duties."

The incident was never mentioned again.

Since the restructuring of health care in the early 1980s, nursing documentation has become increasingly bound to reimbursement. There are urgings to have insurers pay directly for services provided, "tying care to cash." Increasingly, hospitals are being forced to "cost out" how much of each health dollar is dependent upon good or bad nursing care, a trend many hospitals are resisting. Traditionally, nursing care has been budgeted under "room and board" for a hospital stay. DRGs (diagnostic-related groups) have been an impetus for cost-effective research that many nurses have been calling for. For years, it has been estimated that 20 percent of the average hospital budget is allocated for paying nurses, while 75 percent of the services are provided by nurses—a bargain on anybody's ledger.

Such investigations have been a double-edged sword for nurses. There are many who resist reducing the profession to its lowest common denominator—the tasks performed—by shaving off the essence of nursing—human interaction and care giving—because those qualities are so difficult to quantify. Maureen, a pool nurse who floats between floors and units, is among those who feel that the preoccupation with documentation is nothing but another barrier separating her from quality patient contact. There isn't time to do both effectively and still get out on time.

However, if that is the trend in health care, she wants to have her contributions recognized. Recently, a friend of her daughter was hospitalized. Visiting the child at home afterward, her mother showed Maureen the bill. Forty-eight dollars was itemized for dropping an NG tube. One could easily get the impression a physician did that, but she knew it was a nurse. Nowhere was there any indication a nurse had ever touched the child. She thought, If I had one percent for every NG tube I've dropped, I'd be a rich woman.

"Why aren't we fighting for that? It's just another way nursing negates itself. Look who does what in a hospital, Mr. and Ms. Health Consumer take heed: 'I'm the one who changed your dressing. . . . I'm the one who assisted with putting your CVP in, and I'm the one who took it out. . . . I'm the one who put your Foley in. . . . I'm the one who put your NG tube in. . . . I'm the one who was there doing your Swan readings or getting your blood gases or putting ice in your heart for cardiac output monitoring and reading the studies. . . . That's no doctor doing that. Half of them don't even know how to work the machines. I'm generating billable services.'

"People hate to hear that. Money is the last taboo in our profession. The image used to be that we were prostitutes, or that we were in the closet with the doctors. It's always like we have nothing on our little minds but sex. That's because they'd rather we had sex on our minds than, God forbid, money.

"I've actually had an administrator say to me, 'How can you think about money? My God, you're a nurse!' And this was a nursing administrator. Well, I'm a single parent, and I work for a living just like the guy standing in the road waving a flag for Bell Tel, who's been getting paid more than I have for a long time. People say nurses should be paid more because of the shortage and AIDS and everything. Well, lemme tell you, when I hear nurses say they want a raise, I say, 'I don't want a raise—I want profit sharing, honey.'"

When the Joint Commission or the Health Department comes to inspect a hospital—never unannounced—there is always a whirlwind of activity bringing everything up to scratch. Nurses ferociously update their care plans, every other discipline doing likewise with its particular documents. With this burgeoning emphasis on documentation, Maureen has difficulty maintaining the belief that patient care is the most important part of the job. It takes time to give another human being positive regard, but when she's up to her ass in legalities she needs to cover herself for, it's easy to lose sight of the people she came to help. When she makes her initial head-to-toe assessment of patients, she always makes a point of introducing herself. That is often the only meaningful time she spends with those people.

Maureen feels that if she were to work full-time on a med-surg floor, she would have to change her belief system about what nursing is, the caring part of care giving. She has done so on occasion, modifying self-expectations in order to get through certain shifts, giving the minimal amount of herself to get the work done. Something had to give. Unfortunately, the easiest part to give up is human contact. The milk of human kindness is very hard to swallow when you are running very fast.

She'll go down the hall at the end of a shift, knowing she has done more than she can ever remember, knowing she will never accurately recount it all in her nursing notes or in report—and knowing that if she is ever called into a courtroom ten years later, those notes aren't going to do her a damn bit of good—but knowing she has covered herself enough so that the head nurse won't call her at home and complain about it. She can't afford to have administration or her head nurse looking over her shoulder, saying, "Maureen, are you organizing yourself properly? Your care plans are three days overdue. Are you having problems with your paperwork and your time management?" Such judgments get written into her yearly evaluation, becoming a part of her permanent employee record.

She leaves work after such shifts feeling badly about herself because, while she worked herself into a stupor, she wasn't nice to a single person. That's the worst feeling. It's not working over her scheduled hours to get caught up, it's not the paperwork. It's remembering the old man who called out, "Nur—, Nur—" as she sped by his room without a minute to stop because she knew his issues weren't important at that moment. She'd already attended to his bodily needs but literally did not have a minute for kindness.

Kathy's worst experience, in terms of feeling like a humanoid, was an evening shift at her current hospital. On the fourth floor, where she often works, there is a conference room at the end of the hall. The corresponding room on the third floor is a patient room. When she received report for that shift, the day nurse flipped through the Kardex hurriedly, forgetting to include the person in that room. Kathy, jotting notes on her brains, missed the omission.

That was at 3:00 P.M.

At 11:30 P.M., when she sat down to give report, she was feeling good, on top of everything. The shift had flowed smoothly. She'd had a lot of patient-contact time and still felt really thorough. She had a notation for every p.r.n. she'd given, including a follow-up comment on its effects. She knew how many c.c.s she had left in every IV. She was cooking.

Completing report, she stood to leave, pocketbook slung over her shoulder, ready to sashay down the hall, when the oncoming nurse asked, "What about Mr. X?"

"Who?"

"You know." The other RN flipped open the procedure Kardex with the hub of her Scripto, tapping the laminated border. "In 304."

Kathy peered across her shoulder. Sure enough, Mr. X was her patient. Her mouth went dry. She was horrified. Prayers formed in her head. As calmly as possible, she said, "Ah, excuse me just a sec', okay?"

She reached the room at a dead run, shoes squeaking on the tile. She opened the door, tapped the dimmer switch, and crept up to the bed. He was breathing, thank God, in a deep slumber. His vitals were stable. He was dry.

> "God was on my side that night. This man had no meds ordered, no treatments. He had some weird diagnosis like 'sleeping a lot' and was NPO [no food or fluids by mouth]. Still, this man had been seen by nobody for eight hours, maybe sixteen hours. He never woke up and never knew. But he could have been dead in there all shift."

In the clinical realm, diagnostic-related groups fell on floor nurses like a hammer. Because it is more difficult to be admitted, those patients who do make it in are more uniformly impaired than anyone ever envisioned prior to 1983, requiring increased amounts of nursing care.

When Maureen started in nursing, in 1980, she worked on a floor that was next to a step-down unit. This is an area for patients who have been weaned away from intensive care but require greater than average nursing surveillance. Patients would progress from the coronary care unit (CCU) to the medical intensive care unit (MICU) to the step-down unit and, finally, to the floor. It was a steady progression of wellness. At any given time, there was a mix in the degree of care the patient group required. There might be five or six "completes," patients needing total care with hygiene, eating, and movement, while others needed help only with the most taxing efforts. There were also always a few "walkie-talkies" able to take their own baths, feed themselves, and ambulate with a fair degree of certainty. There were actually people who could take medications by mouth in less than ten minutes.

Today there are no more walking wounded, no one in a self-care mode. Many surgeries that would have been admissions in pre-DRG days—things like cataracts, where someone doesn't feel too well for a short spell and then is on his feet again, able to care for himself—aren't seen as often. And those who get admitted are discharged sooner. Patients today are being sent home with IVs and on TPN (total parenteral nutrition, being fed through tubes) and with ventilators. Things that are intimidating to new nurses in ICUs are being taught to family members so they can manage in the home.

The current impetus is to "get'm in and get'm out." Motivation follows money. "Justification" is the buzzword—justifying length of stay for insurers so the hospital gets paid. There are already a few lawsuits popping up around the country exploring the validity of insurance companies dictating treatment cure for patients. The turnover rate is staggering, necessitating more workups. For each admission, Maureen fills out an admission evaluation form, transcribes all orders to medication and treatment Kardexes, starts flow sheets for intake and output (I&O), writes a nursing care plan, a nursing note, and discharge goals.

Because patients are sicker, with less time to heal—for nurses, more work in less time—staff members have had to alter the kinds of things they do. When Maureen works on the floor called "Geri Heaven," where everybody is on Medicare (and DRGs and Medicare are married) it is not uncommon that she will spend three hours just administering medications. Many of the patients are too ill to eat, much less take medicine by mouth. And it's tough getting pills into a nasogastric (NG) tube. When

she crushes many of the new brands of medicine, coated with
filmy tab coverings, she has to tweezer out the tiny, flimsy bits
before mixing them in water so they can be swallowed.

Afterward, it requires lifting some little old lady up, holding
her head, whispering, "C'mon, Mary, a little bit more," while
wanting to kick herself for putting so much water in there—I
mean, my God, it's only ten milliliters, but it's taking her for-
ever!—"C'mon, hon, it's just a *tiny* mouthful. . . ."

Then Maureen repeats the process with Mary's Dilantin for
seizures or her Symmetrel for her parkinsonian tremors. Plus,
Mary is taking these monster horse pills, like Bactrim, for her
urinary tract infection and NSAIDs (nonsteroidal anti-
inflammatory drugs), like Motrin, for her arthritis. The thing about
NSAIDs is that they can cause terrible GI ulcers and are supposed
to be taken with several large glasses of water. But it feels like
most of the patients taking them are eighty years old and can
barely sip. Plus, they have no gag reflex left, so that once Maureen
has macerated the pills to the point where they are able to be
given, it is necessary to lean up real close, wondering, "Gee, did
she get that down?" when, *plugh*, Mary spits them out, spraying
the sheets, Maureen's face, hair, and uniform.

"You are chopping, mixing, dicing, and microwaving meds
because everyone is just so sick. Somebody should do a study
on the effects of microwaving meds. We could be eradicating
their main effects, but it's speedy, it's efficient, and you can
get them in. You've got to get them dissolved enough so that
people can swallow them. Some meds are not crushable, and
when you swish them in water, a lot stick to the side. But if
you put them in a microwave for thirty seconds, you've got
yourself a nice little solution that goes right down—no muss,
no fuss.

"DRGs have done this to me. They've taken away the wellness that gave balance to a floor. I take them as a personal
attack on me getting out on time. I curse DRGs with every
pill I crush."

Karen, an RN since 1975, sees the effects of DRGs in the rapidity of discharges. She has been on the staff of a cardiac rehab floor since 1981. Her title is cardiac nurse educator. She is a slender brunet with a calming demeanor. She does more counseling than anything else, talking with patients who have just had a heart attack or a cardiac problem diagnosed. She makes sure each patient understands his diagnosis, and assists him with finding ways to cope with this intruder in his life.

She assesses each client—his understanding of limitations and expectations, how he is dealing with what is often an abrupt change in his perception of life and, most importantly, what he wants for himself. Then she gives him information that may make it easier to get whatever that is.

At the inception of the program, it was all inpatient, acute-phase work. Because of early discharge dates, the lab has created an active outpatient follow-up group. Pre-DRG, minimum length of stay (LOS) for an uncomplicated inferior MI (myocardial infarction, a heart attack) was two weeks. Patients went through a gradual, fourteen-step program to get ready to go home—first day, bed rest; second day, to bathroom. . . . By discharge day, each patient was stable, with a clear understanding of what he'd gone through and how he could reduce the likelihood of relapse. The program was established as a resource in the community. Karen still hears from many of those people.

Today, an uncomplicated MI goes home in five days. Karen feels lucky if she can get in to *see* them before discharge. It is reflected in those who attend the outpatient program she helps run. People are weaker, sicker, and less informed. It worries her a great deal. What she likes best about her work are the people and the situation in which they meet. She gets to know them very quickly. She approaches them on a topic they are acutely interested in—their health. Mostly patients are in a crisis. It is easy to get past the facade of social encounters, ''how's-the-weather'' sorts of things. There is some of that, but mostly she gets into the marrow of a patient's life right away.

"For every creep you meet, there are plenty of good people. I have a very clear idea of what a strong marriage is because I've seen people and how they can support each other through bad times. It puts things into perspective, just what's really important in this life. It's usually the best they can be."

The outpatient group tries to compensate for what clients missed during abrupt hospitalizations. Participants are involved in a full roster of activities including aerobics classes for people who have been diagnosed with heart disease by positive stress tests. Exercise can reduce coronary heart disease, even when other factors such as diet and weight remain constant. Stationary exercycles and rowing machines are used to enhance cardiopulmonary functioning. Additional teaching and counseling are available to enhance interpersonal functioning.

Most who attend say they leave feeling better.

Other nurses who hear of Karen's work say, "Boy, what a fun job." What they're not seeing is the potential for trouble. They're not seeing the patient on the bike with inoperable coronary artery disease and a 20 percent ejection fraction, who is throwing out PVCs (pre-ventricular contractions) with chest pain, whom she is telling to pedal on, knowing that if he has an MI, she'll be writing out incident reports or giving depositions until the Second Coming. She also knows that by having him ride that bike, when he returns the next day, he will have less discomfort and fewer PVCs, and that within eight weeks they will be gone and he will be walking up hills and stairs. The only way to get him there is to push him through the scary times, the potential danger hovering at all times.

Sometimes that potential is realized. Karen was the only staff member present when a female class member went into cardiac arrest. Karen was the only one to perform CPR for what seemed a long, long time before help arrived. It was a good resuscitation; the woman had good blood gases when brought into the ER.

"In a code, you find out that no matter how many times you're in one, when somebody's giving those IV pushes, everybody's hands are shaking. It's amazing. You realize that everybody is the same."

Throughout the ordeal, sixteen of the woman's classmates stood mutely looking on. For the next class, a few days later, *every*body was there, being very supportive to Karen and each other. It didn't hurt any that the woman's hospital room looked down on the exercise area, and she was able to stand at her window blowing kisses to everyone.

She lived for another year. The night she died, she had been out to dinner with another member of the aerobics class. Before being dropped at home, she had said, "I feel better than I ever have in my entire life."

She went to bed and never awoke.

It took three years of proposal writing and wheedling by Karen's supervisor, a nurse practitioner who started the cardiac lab in 1977, to acquire the space for the exercycles. Then, when DRGs came, somebody got axed and an office was appropriated. Part of what Karen enjoys about her job is being in a small department. She answers to only one person. Her supervisor is very flexible and eager for change. She gets bored fast. Sometimes that can be irritating, but it is never dull. Returning from vacation last year, Karen found the offices empty, rugs rolled up, and the furniture piled in the hall. She had to climb across it to get to a phone, certain the department had fallen to another of the rolling recessions that DRGs have wrought.

"Is there something you want to tell me?" Karen sighed into the receiver when she'd reached her supervisor.

"Don't worry." She laughed. "We're still in business. We had to clear the place out because tomorrow we're starting a seminar for thirty people. Hope you got a lot of rest. See ya."

Paperwork consumes much of Karen's time. The department was always small. DRGs shrank the staff further, while expanding the program. Karen herself was one of those caught in the first round of DRG attrition. The accountants saw that the department wasn't generating enough revenue. Things like inpatient teaching were considered a service and not charged for at that time. The secretary was fired outright. Karen's position was cut back to half-time.

While there is lingering resentment at being considered discardable by the hospital, the new arrangement actually worked nicely into Karen's life. Her first child was born around the same time, and she was able to construct a schedule with a great deal of child-care time.

Karen spent the better part of a week on a paper chase for a man who wished to join the aerobics class. It is necessary to get a physician's approval before someone can attend. Simple, right? Forms are sent out, signed, and returned. Unfortunately, this gentleman had changed physicians, a fact unknown until the first form came back. He'd left his previous doctor under querulous circumstances, and the secretary didn't want to even say who his new physician was. It took eight calls just to get the stress-test results.

Meantime, this man was growing increasingly perturbed about the delays in his joining the class. And he was not shy about letting everyone know it. For Karen, who worked in a CCU before this position, someone arresting is bad, but she finds it even harder dealing with someone who is mad. That's why she never followed an impulse to work in psych nursing, where staff members get cursed out twenty times a day.

He was just a very difficult person to communicate with, unaware of all the extra efforts she made on his behalf, much of it on her own time. There were moments she had to hold her tongue, wanting to lash out herself, "I know you're very ill and need somebody to be angry at, but I'm not particularly looking for the job."

"It was just a bad week for this kind of thing. I had a sick child at home, so I felt torn. I was almost ready to quit because I either had to neglect my job, which I like and feel a certain responsibility for, or I had to neglect my child, who was with my parents, but who was quite sick. I'm lucky because I have my parents as baby-sitters. I don't know how people cope with leaving them with strangers.

"And I'll tell you, there's no support within the system for that frustration. There are a few hospitals that have been starting day care, but this place found fifty billion reasons not to. It continues to show you the regard women have in society as valued professionals. Last year there were something like a hundred bills introduced in Congress about child care, and not one passed. Now that more women are moving into out-of-house work, they are starting to experience what nurses have dealt with for decades. Businesses are starting to deal with the problem, like there's all this talk about 'the Mommy Track,' so maybe something will change.

"Luckily, this position is flexible. If I had to leave for an emergency, I could. But that would leave my supervisor to handle it by herself. I guess she could call off the class. That would mean calling twenty-five type-A personalities and telling them their class has been canceled. Sure!"

Powerlessness is a recurring theme in the conversations of staff nurses. Hospital nursing administrations are structured on the military model, decisions filtering down through echelons of authority. Many nurses feel they are far more committed to protecting the institution than any individual nurse. Maureen sees other groups doing a much better job of protecting their own. Social workers are always drawing the wagons around. They'll cover one another's butts ad infinitum and forever. As do dietitians, pharmacists, and housekeeping. God knows, doctors do it like it's a religious reflex. But in nursing, administratively, at least, she feels there is little support for nurses.

She had an instance when a husband complained that he'd asked Maureen for some Alka-Seltzer for his wife. They were an elderly couple, mid-seventies, both very ill. Each was traumatized by the fact that the other had cancer. She, being the sickest at that point, now had intestinal gas that escalated into vomiting. He kept running in and out with exclamations and updates of what was going on.

Basically, the problem was that his wife didn't have an order to receive that medication, and the pharmacy didn't have it in stock anyway. So Maureen was waiting for the on-call oncology fellow to phone in from home to get an order for the woman to have *some*thing when her husband went off like a beanbag, screaming about how incompetent the staff was, how his wife's doctor was going to hear about this, how heads would roll. Finally, the fellow called, and Maureen got an order for a Compazine injection.

The next day, the husband complained to the head nurse about how mean and vicious Maureen had been. He said he'd had to beg for her to pay any attention to him, and it was only after repeated pleas that she responded by giving his wife anything. He wasn't a very reliable historian, his story changing a bit in detail with each retelling. In actuality, it wasn't even her he'd originally asked. He'd spoken with another nurse while she was at dinner. The other nurse was built like Maureen—not as heavy, but she could see how, *maybe*, he could have mistaken them. She didn't think she would have but was willing to give him the benefit of the doubt. At any rate, he was fixated it was Maureen. . . .

Still, Maureen had to deal with this. She was called up to the director of nursing's office, where the DON and the pool head nurse wanted to know what happened. She found herself having to defend herself and calling in other staff members who were present to corroborate events. Luckily, the other regular floor nurses there said, "He's not telling the truth. That's not what happened at all. Maureen wasn't even there for most of the incident."

One of his points was that Maureen had given an IM injection to his wife while she was standing up, failing to mention that this was his wife's request. He accused Maureen of having "stabbed" his wife with the needle.

"Well, he was *so* upset, that it *must*'ve happened that way," the head nurse said. As if human beings don't get upset, especially when sick, and out of proportion to any actual incident.

"One of the big problems in nursing is that everything above the staff level is administrative. You have to make a decision whether you're a nurse or an administrator, who doesn't do anything resembling nursing. Even head nurses are totally management. It strikes me as a means to keep nurses from organizing, to keep us powerless.

"Where is the staff nurse's advocate? We've asked for a mechanism for taking complaints upward in the chain of command. With the reverse there's no problem; that route works very well, thank you. But if you tell your head nurse a problem, you don't know where it goes.

"Three months later, when the nursing administrator is making her rounds and you mention your concern to her, she says, 'Oh, gee, I didn't know. I would have answered if I knew. I respond to all the complaints I *receive.*'

"There is this attitude that you're to blame because you didn't personally hand deliver a note. However, if you go around your head nurse, you're 'bucking the chain of command' or, worse, advocating a union. Try that and they'll pull out the holy water and the garlic, and drive a crucifix through your heart."

At a meeting of the nursing staff called to address such issues, the presiding VP wasn't grasping the staff's concerns. Kathy raised her hand in response to a question on the floor: "What is it administration can do to help you feel that your input is valued?"

"All we want," Kathy began, "is something that would give us a little more power. Like if we had a group that would just be *for* the nurses—staff nurses—*of* the nurses, *by* the nurses. . . . Not a union, just a support group. Not for more money, but for a voice."

"But you have one," he said. "There's a task force."

"No, not a group assigned by you guys," she responded, echoed by grumbles of agreement. Kathy has watched administration invite select employees—people who will be *honored* to be chosen—to form groups to come to the opinions they want reached. Then, if conflicts arise, they can say, "Oh, but your employee group said, 'Blah, blah, blah. . . . ' We had a group of you in here, and that's what they decided."

"Well, what do you want a voice for when you can knock on my door anytime?"

"If I come and knock on your door, you're gonna be very paternal and say, 'Oh, that's nice . . .' and when I leave, you'll put it aside and forget about it. I'm sure my sole problem won't rush to the top of your list. But if there's fifty or sixty of us who sign a petition that says that we feel a certain way, you're not gonna be as likely to ignore it. It would give us a little power."

"Well," the VP began uneasily, "what do you mean by power?"

Had she not been so hungry and tired, she probably wouldn't have spoken. But she looked at him and said, "Power. You know what power is, because you have it. It's those of us who don't have it who want to find out about it. We're not exactly sure what it is, but we know we don't have it. It's like love: if you have it, you don't have to ask, and if you don't have it, you just know you're missing something very important."

"Needless to say, he didn't much care for this little scene from *Norma Rae*. I guess because we had female apparatus on our bodies that he thought we didn't have minds, too. It seemed to astound him.

"We still haven't gotten the group."

It is not unusual for a hospital staff nurse to be asked to be a part of things she is not introduced to, is not a party to, and with which she does not agree. But the nurse is there. It falls on her, and she is expected to deal with it.

Maureen was charge nurse on oncology, evening shift. One of the patients—Evelyn O., a married sixty-two-year-old Caucasian female—had a tumor in her neck at her carotid artery. She had gone through a moderate amount of chemotherapy, which she found repulsive. After consultation with family and physician, she decided to forgo further treatment. She considered herself a realist and resolved to live out her life "in a natural manner" and face a peaceful, dignified death.

To assist in this, to assure someone was with her at the end, she had private-duty nurses on day and evening shifts, frequent supportive visits from her husband—himself a physician, a hospital department director—and during the nights, the companionship of her longtime housekeeper.

It was known on admission that she was on borrowed time. She had already experienced two near bleed outs. Her standing orders were firm: she was not to be disturbed in any way. Because any movement could precipitate a rupture, she was not to be changed or turned, no hygienic measures performed. One of her personal requests was that no "invasive procedures" be done on her. To comply, not even a urinary catheter was inserted. In consequence, she regularly urinated on herself, but not even the disposable absorbent pads beneath her were to be replaced.

Maureen found it all very offensive.

"I had a problem with that. Like, why bring her to us and make us watch this horrible thing happen? I mean, she's a stranger to me. It's a queer thing, socially, to ask of someone. If you want to die 'peacefully,' can't you do it at home? Can't you have a nurse come in who agrees to do that? Can't you find some 'meaningful other' who agrees to witness your death with you and not intervene, rather than put this on somebody whose whole job is to help save and improve the quality of life?"

At about 10:45, Mrs. O.'s agency nurse came out to Maureen and asked if it would be all right if she left early. Mrs. O. was resting quietly, and her housekeeper would be in soon. Her attending physician had left less than a half hour earlier. No problems were foreseen.

Maureen knew the private-duty nurse and trusted her judgment. After peeking in on Mrs. O., Maureen said, ''You go ahead. It's okay. I'll keep an eye on her until the housekeeper gets here.''

''Thanks.''

Maureen was tidying up the medication cart, making last-minute Kardex notations, when Mrs. O.'s call bell rang. Maureen entered the room and witnessed her first arterial bleed.

Maureen had always heard that exsanguination was a rapid process; you became listless, unconscious, and were gone. That was nothing like this. Blood was on the ceiling, on the closet to the right, on the wall to the left. It was slamming against the wall at the foot of the bed. As Maureen approached, it slammed into her face.

''Do you want me to suction you?'' she gasped.

Mrs. O. didn't respond, staring directly into Maureen's face, blinking. Blood gurgled out of her trach, out the ulcerated site on her neck, out her nose, her mouth. She gripped Maureen's hand.

''Oh, dear God,'' Maureen implored. ''Won't you let me help you? What can I do?''

Mrs. O.'s free hand reached up to wipe her nose and mouth. She lifted it to eye level and stared at the blood on her fingers.

''And you're a witness to this. You're an absolute witness. Here she is having her supposed 'meaningful moment' that she'd planned for and orchestrated grandly with her husband and housekeeper. . . . Well, lemme tell you, they did a lousy job of it because I was the meaningful other who shared her death with her. And I'd known her for all of five minutes.

''Her blue eyes looked into mine for the full twenty minutes it took her to die. She held my hand. She was a little woman.

You wouldn't think there was that much blood in a body. I can still feel it splashing in my face.

"And I wasn't allowed to do anything."

Word flashed like wildfire throughout the floors: something freakish on oncology. Soon faces appeared at the door, environmental service and maintenance staff—two, three in a vertical pattern. Then the door opened wider to accommodate the overflow. Maureen caught first sight of them in the dresser mirror. She waved them away behind her back, trying to focus on Mrs. O.'s spiritual needs, praying with her, encouraging relaxation, calmness.

"It's okay, Evelyn. I'm here for you. Just let go. . . ."

She attempted to ignore the whispers and nervous gasps, her indignation rising, hoping to assist as a peaceful presence as Evelyn went from what Maureen believes was this world to the next, while they gawked like this was a freak show. It was difficult enough trying to share a private, intimate moment with this woman in this scene without also having an audience.

She also tried to juggle logistics in her mind. It was eleven o'clock, and the next shift would be coming in at eleven-thirty. She had to organize information for report. She still had meds she hadn't given out. And there was blood all over the room, blood all over her body; it felt like being in a war. She knew she'd have to buy a new uniform. Then there was the body to be cleaned and transported.

"You've got all these things going on. I was in a religious crisis because there's a part of me that believes in the right to live as you wish, and that somebody should be there with you who understands your personal feelings about dying and your right to do so. I was in a nursing crisis because I've got a woman exsanguinating before me and I'm allowing it, which is against everything I've been taught and believe in personally. Then there was the floor management crisis.

"On top of it all, her housekeeper arrived and started

shrieking like a banshee. Then she needed comforting. I understood her trauma—she'd known this woman a long time. I don't know what she expected when she signed on for this duty, but, jeez, this just turned into a scene out of *Gone With The Wind*: 'I don't know *nuttin'* 'bout no death with *dignity*!'

"Now, after three years, I can be calm about it. But at the time, she was screaming in the corner, the maintenance contingent was skulking at the door, and along with everything else, I needed to document all that happened in some fashion. Sometimes I think there's nothing more insulting in life than having to write it all down afterward in a nursing note."

Afterward, Maureen felt like she needed to be debriefed, but nobody wanted to talk about it. Night shift wanted to get in and evening shift wanted to get out. She tried to discuss it with the evening supervisor, who shrugged it off.

"Well, Maureen, you know it comes with the territory. If you can't handle it . . ."

She didn't sleep well for three weeks. She would return to her apartment nightly and sit in the dark. She wondered how safe a practitioner she could be, going through shifts stunned, psychically traumatized. None of the people who made it so important not to touch Mrs. O. ever contacted her. Dr. O. never called to say, "I understand you were with my wife. . . ." The attending physician never stopped by. Pastoral care had gone on retreat.

"In our hospital, we have this nice nursing philosophy that talks about our humanity, our caring. It's posted in all the nursing stations. Yet, in the busy profession we're in, when something very human and catastrophic happens, you're not allowed to respond to it in a natural, human way. They act like it didn't happen to you. There's this 'tough it out or get out' attitude. Like you should give up your career because something happened that was out of the ordinary and you reacted to it.

"Not one person ever said, 'Gee, Maureen, good job. You

did what you were supposed to do' or 'Gosh, that must've been a tough one.' Not even a, 'Hey, lemme pass your meds for ya.'

"To this day, that astounds me."

There are days when Kathy decides to be nice to herself, to take that full half-hour lunch, off the floor where she can sit with her feet stationary, not inhaling her food, not catching up on progress notes or care plans or flow sheets, but like a normal person, relaxing and maybe even conversing about something other than nursing. Sometimes there's a nagging notion in the back of her mind that perhaps this isn't a good idea; she has looked at whom she is working with, whom she'll be signing patients off to during this foray. Maybe it's an FTN (foreign-trained nurse) who understands only a little English, or someone who is so stupid Kathy wonders how she ever could have passed her state boards, or someone who is a tad glassy-eyed—possibly because she is not clear from the night before or possibly because she is currently using drugs and spent an inordinate amount of time in the bathroom all morning. But her gut instincts get overruled, and she goes anyway.

Kathy returned from lunch on such a day once while working in Pittsburgh. Pushing through the fire doors, she heard the shrieks of a co-worker and immediately thought someone must have coded or hung himself in a Posey.

"My God, Kathy, your patient is choking!"

Great for the digestion. Kathy ran down to the room where an obese, gagging woman sat in bed, hands to her throat, crimson-faced, legs thrashing, while her visitors thumped her on the back. Kathy stood in the door, slack-jawed, taking in the scene, as the family shouted, "*Do* something! Do something, quick. Please, oh, dear God, help her!"

This was before the introduction of the Heimlich maneuver. Not knowing what to do, Kathy grasped the suction catheter, having to fight the panic-stricken woman to get it into her mouth. She heard the suction suck go *phwet*! and cease making sound. She pulled back, but it wouldn't budge.

One family member kept yelping for Kathy to do something. Another was reassuring the patient while attempting to restrain her hands. He kept losing his grip, and hands would fly up into Kathy's face trying to push her away. Kathy was yanking the catheter without luck, putting her body weight behind it, feeling sweat streams flow, her hands slippery, grip sliding, thinking she was going to lose this lady and wondering where the hell her reinforcements were when, *thunk*, out plunked the catheter, a massive chunk of kielbasa stuck to its quivering tip.

The family must have brought it to her for lunch. It was huge. There was no way it could have been swallowed. Kathy guessed she must have been chewing it pronged to a fork when somebody told her a joke, and she inhaled the whole damn thing. As soon as she saw the woman was all right, gulping down mouthfuls of air, Kathy's laughter began. Deep, rolling, uncontrollable spasms. It was the only time in her career she collapsed in laughter—giggles, guffaws, snorts, and cackles. Right across the patient's lap, her feet and legs off the floor, tears coming down her cheeks.

''It was partly because it was funny, and partly because I'd been afraid she was going to die on me. It was such a relief. But I was laughing, and the family was getting really annoyed. I couldn't stop. I was hurting this lady's legs. Somebody ran down the hall and got my head nurse. She came in, and the kielbasa was on the end of the catheter with the suction still hissing.

''By now the family is *really* mad, the patient is aghast, and I'm roaring. As imperiously as she could, my head nurse picked me off the bed and said, 'Kathy, come down to my office. *Now*!'

''I followed her down there. She shut the door, and we both just laughed our asses off.''

7

"Hopefully Some Listening"

Psychiatric Floors

Suzanne double-checks the assignment sheet, jotting "NCP due" next to patient names. It seems that everybody's nursing care plan is out of date. Three of her four primary patients need revisions. Rose, her head nurse, made it firmly clear in report that care-plan revisions are a priority. State inspectors are due at the end of the week. All paperwork has to be up to date by Wednesday. Suzanne, scheduled to attend a psychiatric nursing conference, is delighted she'll be off the two days of the inspection.

The hospital is a renowned private psychiatric facility situated on ample acreage. There are several buildings, sprawling lawns and gardens, playing fields, tennis courts, a pool, and a dense surrounding timberline enhancing the sense of privacy as advertised in the hospital's brochure.

Along with Rose and Suzanne, the 7:00 A.M. floor shift consists of another staff nurse, Penny—who is "doubling back," having worked the 3:00 to 11:30 shift last night—and three psych techs. Psychiatric technicians (PTs) are employed by the nursing department. In the chain of command, a PT is the mental health equivalent of a nursing assistant. However, many PTs have diverse backgrounds, often with greater educational credentials than the RNs who supervise their work. Still, PTs practice under the umbrella of the staff nurse's license and are accountable to her.

Rose leans against the chart rack, phone in hand. She has been trying to wrangle someone from the maintenance department into repairing the nurses' station wall clock, which has been hanging by exposed wires for months.

"I *have* filed the forms," she says, tapping her foot. "At least twice."

Two psych techs, one each from the night and morning shifts, count sharps. Anything patients might use to harm themselves with is confiscated on admission. Razors, scissors, glass perfume bottles, aerosol cans, etc. The owner is able to sign his or her belongings out when needed unless he or she is on one of three levels of self-injury precautions. Then a staff member must supervise its use.

Everything is accounted for except the razor hidden by a patient yesterday, which the staff had been unable to locate, even after a room-to-room search.

Normally on a Monday when she hasn't worked the weekend before—and assuming the other nurse has—Suzanne will pour medications, allowing the nurse with a more consistent presence on the unit to assume charge duties. This morning, however, Penny requested meds. She wanted a task that would remove her from the patients for a while, something structured and concrete. The medication room, a converted closet barely large enough for two people to stand in, is just what she needs.

Flipping through the med Kardex, Penny sips her second cup of coffee. When she and Suzanne divvied up the assignments, Penny had hoped to avoid the morning community meeting, but Rose insisted her presence was mandatory. Penny knew the meeting was going to be one of those patient bitch sessions where no matter what the staff did, it was wrong. It had been a bad weekend. During the course of both Sunday shifts, a patient had attempted to burn a nurse with a cigarette and three patients spent time in LDS (locked-door seclusion). One of them, Pam, was still cooling her heels in there.

Penny stretches and massages her scalp through auburn curls, trying to shake off her lassitude. She hadn't left the building until well after midnight, documenting all the p.r.n. ("as needed") meds she'd given and conferring with the nursing supervisor and resident on call. The unit's anxiety remained palpable when she returned this morning. Some shifts she can just feel it. She's tempted to add extra doses to everyone's meds just to calm the place down.

"It'll just be you and me." Rose leans into the med room to quickly confer with Penny. Keeping each other apprised of their location is something Rose tries to inculcate in her staff. "Katy and Allen are taking the patient group down for breakfast. I wanted to get as many of them off as possible today."

The floor employs a five-step "patient responsibility level." It is used as a gauge of individual patient privileges. On the lowest level, patients are restricted to the floor. On the highest, they may leave the floor unescorted and take unaccompanied trips off the hospital grounds, though this is rarely done anymore because insurance reviewers will disallow payment for those days, employing the argument that if a patient can be off hospital property, then they can be discharged.

Most of the patients are on level three, meaning they can leave the unit in a group escorted by a staff member. The limit is five patients per staff member. With staff turnovers lately, it's been hard for Rose to get more than five off the unit for each meal, leading to endless complaints. She hates it when so many decisions that should be based upon the therapeutic needs of individual patients are swallowed in the shadows of short staffing.

"Ken is in with Harry C., so he can shave," she continues. Harry is one of the patients who lost control yesterday and threatened suicide. "I'll be out on the unit. Suzanne's down at ECT."

"Okay," Penny nods, dropping pills into a soufflé cup.

Electroconvulsive therapy, popularly called "shock treatment," is offered each Monday, Wednesday, and Friday morning. An RN needs to accompany each patient who goes, transporting them in a wheelchair to the treatment room and back. Luckily, there's only one patient on the unit receiving it. When there are two or three, it can be a real juggling act for Rose to meet the schedule.

Rose picks up a clipboard with a sheet listing each patient name and room number. Beside each name are timed blocks where staff can record the location and coded activity of the patient. On "patient rounds," everyone is checked on at least hourly. If the patient is on a *close observation status*, such as *arson precautions* or *elopement precautions*, then they are checked at least every fifteen minutes. There are a series of self-injury precautions also. On SIP-I patients are checked on at least every fifteen minutes and only leave the floor if accompanied by a staff member. SIP-II restrictions include the above plus being limited to common areas within staff eyesight at all times, even sleeping in the lounge. On SIP-III, the status of Harry C. this morning, patients have a nursing staff member within arm's reach at all times, even when using the bathroom or sleeping.

The unit is a "general" unit accepting patients with any psychiatric diagnosis from schizophrenia to panic attacks. The treatment tempo is quicker than it was when Rose took over as head nurse since insurance regulations force quicker discharges. There are a maximum of twenty-two patients on the unit. Ten being off at breakfast, she wanders down the hallway to the lounge, where several are eating breakfast from trays held on laps.

"I just love these little picnics, Rose," one of the adolescent patients says sarcastically. His privilege level would allow him to leave the unit only with a staff group.

"Well," says Rose, jotting her initials next to his name, turning to proceed down the hall. "I guess tomorrow you'll be awake early enough to get your name on the breakfast group list."

"If you snooze, you lose," says Heather, another adolescent.

A week ago they were a couple. The staff had to set limits to keep them from petting every time they got a chance. This week they are sniping at each other at every opportunity.

In the seclusion room, Pam is practicing ballet stances until she sees Rose peering through the observation window. Pam is wearing only a hospital gown and panties, the maximum clothing allowed to someone in LDS.

"You gonna feed me sometime today, Warden?"

"We'll be in to do a break before community meeting," Rose answers through the door.

"I have to pee, too."

"As soon as we have enough staff."

The rule is that at least two staff members be present whenever a seclusion break is done, be it for meals, meds, bathroom, or assessment.

"What's the matter, Rose, 'fraid I'm gonna wrestle you to the ground?" Pam laughs.

"As soon as we have enough staff," Rose repeats flatly. Actually, Rose finds female patients scarier than males, more apt to attack. Her most frightening experience was at the hands of a female patient who had set a fire in her room. Luckily, she had set the blaze in the bathtub, and it was quickly dampened. Of course, there were smoke and an alarm, and the fire department arrived. In the midst of this, Rose had foolishly attempted to place the woman in seclusion without backup. The woman was almost six feet tall, compared with Rose's five-foot-two frame.

"You simply have to go in," Rose had informed her indignantly.

"You can't make me," the woman had said. And she was right. She grabbed Rose and started to choke her, glaring down into Rose's reddening face. Throughout the scuffle, Rose knew help would arrive within minutes, but she learned just how long a minute could be.

"Am I gonna be able to go to community meeting?" Pam inquires.

Morning community meeting is a gathering of all patients and most of the staff present. This includes attending and resident psychiatrists, social workers, activity therapists, medical and nursing students. It is meant to be a place for dealing with any problems on the hall, airing grievances in a constructive manner, and patient self-governance. Like any group, it gives rise to interpersonal conflict and personality displays. It is the basis for what is termed a "therapeutic milieu," where those behaviors that led to hospitalization come into play, allowing the staff to help patients devise more productive methods of dealing with others.

"That hasn't been decided yet," Rose says. Rose feels the milieu therapy on this hall is the best she has ever seen. Too often, the psychiatrists who administer a hall are absentee landlords, preoccupied with their outpatient practices. Here they are very involved, capable, and committed to supporting the milieu concept.

"Well, I'd *better* be," Pam haughtily informs her. "I intend to tell everybody in that room just what a bunch of incompetent assholes the people working here are."

Arriving at her office, Debbie receives a quick report from the day-shift nursing supervisor about events over the weekend. She is not surprised about all the acting out on Rose's unit. Adele Y., a patient recently discharged from that unit, had committed suicide last week. She was an older woman, well liked by patients and staff. She'd gone down to the river, filled her pockets with rocks, and jumped in. She was submerged for a long time, her body wedged between bridge pilings. What made it worse for the patients was the way they found out. One of them had called her at home to invite her to lunch. A police officer, searching the house for a suicide note, answered the phone.

Debbie has worked for this institution for over fifteen years, as a staff nurse, a head nurse, an evening supervisor, and, since receiving her master's degree in adult psychiatric nursing, as a clinical specialist for one of the buildings. Each building houses a variety of specialized units. In Debbie's building, there are a short-term hall where patients stay less than a month, a geriatric hall, an adolescent hall, and a chemical dependence hall. Rose's intermediate-stay hall is on the third floor.

''Clin spec'' is a position Debbie is happy to hold, well worth the nine years of education it took her to get here. It's a fluid position, changing with the needs of the halls over time. One of her responsibilities is helping the staff deal with the emotional turmoil created by the work. The job can create a lot of emotional baggage for staff people, sometimes steamer trunks full. Her own first dealings with suicide were very painful. She had been a nurse for three years and in psych for only one. She was working on a long-term unit. The woman was someone Debbie had worked with for most of that year, and she was the one who found her.

Mrs. V. was an older woman, hospitalized for depression, but she also had a strong hysterical bent. It was her custom to lie down for an hour or so after dinner. She specifically approached two other patients requesting they wake her up at 6:45. Each assured her they would and promptly forgot.

There was to be a party on the hall that evening for a younger female patient who was being discharged. Private psych hospitals, particularly on long-term halls, are highly ritualistic about anyone leaving, be they patient or staff. ''Termination'' can be discussed for days or weeks before the fact: the impact on the milieu, covert or overt messages conveyed. For most people, it may be the closest they will ever come to experiencing celebrity status, with all the attendant-focused attention.

Debbie was doing 7:00 P.M. rounds checks when she discovered Mrs. V., slack-jawed, in her room. She'd overdosed on Darvon, with an allergy to aspirin, probably not knowing that Darvon contained salycitic acid. To this day, Debbie is convinced that it was intended as a manipulative gesture—Mrs. V.'s desire to be found in a semi-comatose state, thus stealing the spotlight from the girl who was leaving—and that when Mrs. V.

awoke in some afterlife, she was more surprised than anybody.

When she found Mrs. V. unresponsive, Debbie panicked. She ran for the phone instead of initiating CPR. It took her a long time afterward to work through that breach of appropriate sequence, the guilt suction pulling her back, again and again, to the thought that had she immediately started CPR, Mrs. V. might have lived. Despite the fact that when resuscitation was started, her lungs were already squishing, her jaw stiffening, her body cooled. She was very dead.

After the fruitless attempts to revive, after the pronouncement of death, the staff called an emergency community meeting—gathering together the ragged therapeutic circle in the community room while Mrs. V. was carried on a stretcher out a back door to a freight elevator—and started the bitter task of working it through with the patients, the shock, regret, rage, and sadness. Throughout it, Debbie felt she was doing reasonably well, numbly functional while mouthing the appropriate phrases. She was still of the selfless frame of mind: the nurse is the professional and doesn't have feelings of her own; onward Christian soldiers!

The next day, a patient stopped her and asked, "How are you doing? You didn't look so good last night."

"Why do you say that?"

"I've never seen anyone as white as you were still standing up."

"It really hit home. . . . I guess it was about that time that I began to incorporate the notion that nurses do, in fact, have feelings, and that it's okay to share some of those feelings—that it's how you go about sharing and what you decide to share that you're accountable for rather than being accountable for having the feelings, particularly negative feelings. There was a part of me that was very angry. I felt like, 'How could you do this to me, after all the effort I put into you?' "

On her desk, Debbie finds a note from Rose asking that she attend the unit's morning meeting.

The seclusion room is equipped with a sound transmitter, the receiver on a desk in the nurses' station. It allows staff an extra method for monitoring the safety of whoever has been secluded. Penny was able to overhear Rose and Pam speaking. She wishes Pam's physician would just discharge the woman. God knows, it's been discussed enough in treatment team meetings. Pam refuses to take the medications he prescribes, refuses to participate in any of the unit activities or groups. She is constantly trying to pit patients against staff and each other.

Her primary therapist is one of the residents Penny has little respect for, refusing to diagnose Pam for what she is. Her formal diagnosis is "major depression." But she's borderline, by any other name, and everybody knows it. Borderline personality disorder is a controversial diagnosis, and therapists are reluctant to label anyone such. But the behavior described by the term is well known to all who work in psychiatric settings. The person is usually intelligent, self-dramatizing, manipulatively seductive, and prone to abrupt mood swings. Self-mutilation with a razor or by burning oneself is common.

What the unit went through the previous evening certainly was a clear-cut case of the borderline domino effect—one person causing problems for the whole hall. Pam was an ace, getting everything churning, everyone seething with "Help me! Help me!" tension. When not crying hysterically, she was yelling and cursing, jabbing emotional sore spots, and seeking allies. As is often the case on an inpatient unit, the issues Pam was able to ignite could be reduced to matters of trust and control: Can we be certain the staff will protect us? Who's in charge here? Who are these new staff people? The recent spate of turnovers and use of agency nurses to fill staffing gaps have given her lots of opportunity to act out.

She began by intimating that the adolescent patients had drugs hidden on the unit, which had several of the older patients quite anxious. Then, she quietly alerted the more timid patients that a male patient, Harry C., was gay and HIV-positive, facts not even known to all the staff, which fed their feelings of being expendable and excluded. Naturally, having this information broadcast enraged Harry, who had been assured by his psychiatrist that his confidentiality would be maintained. Then she hid the razor, informing everyone that the staff was too stupid to find it. When placed on lounge confinement to be closely observed lest she get the razor and start slicing herself, she broke her glasses, threatening to cut herself with them.

When informed she would have to take a "time-out" to calm herself in the quiet room, she threw her pocketbook at a staff member, cursing him volubly. The quiet room is what seclusion is termed when the room is unlocked. Depending upon the degree of disruption a patient exhibits, he or she is given a choice—voluntarily remove yourself, the door remaining unlocked, or the staff will place you in the room, and the door will remain locked until you exhibit improved self-control.

Naturally, Pam refused; where's the drama in taking time to collect oneself peacefully? The scene then escalated into a struggle and an "All staff call," an emergency PA broadcast to summon as many nursing staff as are available to a unit to quell violence. After attempts to bite staff, she was placed in restraints, screaming all the way.

Afterward all the other borderlines, in sympathy or competition, began grumbling in suicidal tones. Then somebody eloped. The HIV-positive patient broke a vase and threatened to cut his throat, landing him on SIP-III with a staff member remaining within arm's length at all times, which meant a psych tech had to be pulled from another unit. Another patient returned from a tense family outing and also lost control. He was someone Penny is fond of, a normally quiet, neat, sweet guy. He's someone Penny would use to judge the intensity of the hall's tension level. He just absorbed everybody else's anxiety and went off, like a puppy losing control, winding up in the other LDS room. Just your basic nightmare Sunday evening shift.

All this with just three staff people—Penny and two psych techs—who were still responsible for the normal functioning of the unit: getting people to activities, giving out medications, getting care plans up to date, assessing and documenting everyone's functioning level, gathering and giving report. Amid this, Penny got into a conflict with one of the psych techs. He wanted to move Pam into an unlocked quiet room sooner than Penny thought was warranted. The dispute became a question of position versus experience and education, Allen having several more years in the field than Penny and studying for his doctorate in psychology. The conversation became so heated that eventually the evening supervisor became involved. For her, the decision was easy:

"We'll go with Penny's decision because she's the charge nurse."

"Fine, why not?" The tech got all sulky afterward. "Nurses—why the hell do they ask your opinion if they're just gonna do whatever they want anyway?"

"I think there's some validity to that. I certainly want input for decisions, but the buck stops with the nurse who makes or okays it. It's my license that's on the line—he practices on my license. His misjudgment could cost me my career. . . .

"He got real quiet, and I could tell he was pissed. It bothered me in the sense that I don't like conflict. I like to get along with people I work with. But it pissed me off, too, because the last thing I needed on such a stressful night was to worry about how he was doing.

"Later in the shift, we were able to talk about it and resolve it. You have to. You have to be able to work as a team, to be able to count on other staff being there for you, as you are for them."

Debbie arrives on the hall a few minutes before the meeting is to start. On spring mornings like this, with the hospital's pink and white dogwoods in bloom, it is often stunning to enter one of the units and see patients sitting about in sour silence. One sits staring at the wall, occasionally swatting at nothing. Another, Andrew, a bonds trader admitted for depression, complains about having nothing to do.

"What level are you on, Andy?" Debbie asks. She has known him throughout three admissions.

"Five," he says. This would allow him to leave the unit unaccompanied at will.

"It's beautiful out," she says. "You could go for a walk. It's really gorgeous out."

"What's the use?" he scoffs.

She thinks of it as Debbie's Springtime Depression Scale. Her feeling about nursing is that it has never let her down. She is one of the few nurses she knows who gladly admits to liking nursing. *Psych* nursing, that is.

> "What I like about psych nursing is that the majority of people go into remission or they get better or something quote 'positive' happens. I think I have an ability to listen to people, to be able to help them sort out and identify problems and alternatives. I have my own enthusiasms for living, and I don't give up on people if they are hopelessly depressed or very crazy or just out-and-out bastards."

It took Debbie awhile as a staff nurse to understand that psychiatric illnesses were similar to diabetes in terms of being somewhat controllable and going into remission phases. Just as a brittle diabetic will end up rehospitalized, so too will many psych patients. Her treatment goal is to help people cope with a chronic illness, to get them strong and stable, with as solid a support system as can be mustered, before letting them go out on their own.

It took an equal amount of time to realize that all her *wanting* a patient to get better wasn't going to do it. The first couple of schizophrenics whom she spent eighteen or more months working with only to have them return six months after discharge were major blows to her self-esteem. God, but she used to take so much home with her. Today about the most she takes home are the numerous journals that pile up on her desk.

In the community room, two of the techs are being helped by patients to pull chairs into the standard group circle. Debbie prefers to enter such meetings "cold," without staff input, wanting to observe the group dynamic as it unfolds. But Rose waves her into the office, where a dispute is in progress between Pam's therapist, Dick—who insists she be allowed to attend the meeting—and the nursing staff, who feel this would be counter-therapeutic.

"She was in restraints yesterday for trying to bite and kick staff," Penny is explaining.

"Well, sure—after she was dragged into a seclusion room," Dick interrupts. The service chief, Dick's immediate supervisor, stands on the fringe of the group, observing without comment.

Penny fills the narrow passage to the med room, legs apart in battle pose, lips tight. "The staff tried to let her out twice during the night, and each time she stated she had the razor hidden where she could get it," she responds. "The point in her being secluded was to protect her."

Maintaining safety is in large part a nursing responsibility. It often falls to nurses to be "the bad guys," the limit setters. When someone is restricted to the unit, nursing does it, when violence is confronted and quelled, nursing does it.

"Penny, I can't believe you couldn't do a better job of helping her control herself." Dick slaps his palm against his side.

"Maybe that's because you weren't here."

Debbie can see this is escalating to the sarcasm stage.

"Maybe if I was, this all could have been handled better," Dick says.

"Oh, no doubt that would have made all the difference."

"Ah, excuse me, folks—" Debbie tries to cut in, overrun by Dick.

"Why wasn't I called?"

"You were called," Penny insists. "I left messages on your machine."

"Well, I didn't get them," he says accusingly.

Penny shrugs, palms heavenward in a what-the-hell-does-*that*-mean? gesture.

It's Debbie's guess that what is being discussed has nothing to do with the real issue here, which she sees as a new resident, halfway through his first psych placement, attempting to establish his authority. It's a common phenomenon: first there is a "honeymoon phase," when the new doctor is very dependent upon staff nurses to learn the system. After gaining some footing, most attempt to establish a sense of professional identity, to stake out personal terrain, often getting into power struggles. Then again, some people are just jerks.

"I think the point right now is what do we do next?" Rose interrupts, redirecting the conversation, the SC nodding. "The meeting starts in two minutes."

"What about letting the group decide?" Debbie interjects quickly, before too much ego gets invested in either side.

The issues Debbie finds most draining are always staff issues—nursing issues, interdepartmental issues, interpersonal issues with therapists. Very rarely are they patient issues.

When she was a head nurse, the things she disliked most were conflicts with therapists. Once a patient came to her and said, "I'm paying for my hospitalization out of my own pocket. I've been here three weeks and only seen my therapist twice. What can I do about it?"

It was an uncomfortable position. Debbie knew this psychiatrist habitually didn't see patients. Debbie had even complained about it to the service chief, but she got nowhere.

"You need to confront her about it," she said, realizing the absurdity of the comment; how can you confront someone when you can't find her? "I'll also let her know that you and I had this conversation. If you don't get any satisfaction, you always have the option to see the service chief about it.''

The patient tried confrontation, without improvement. She informed Debbie of this a week later. Debbie then reminded her of the option of meeting with the service chief when the woman remarked, ''Debbie, you don't understand. . . . I know my discharge date is being discussed, and my doctor told me in the team meeting that she was the only one who was in favor of my being discharged. Everybody else, including the service chief, was for keeping me for long-term treatment.''

Debbie was stumped. It was a lie. It was blackmail. She had attended all the discharge meetings herself. The woman was in for depression. Because she started on an antidepressant and felt substantially better, all agreed she would soon be able to leave.

Debbie asked for a three-way meeting with the service chief, the therapist, and herself. The therapist distorted all that had been said, maintaining the patient was delusional, which was complete fabrication. The service chief resolved the meeting by stressing a consensus agreement. ''Well, no one disputes that she has improved and is ready for discharge, correct?'' Within a week, the patient was gone, the larger issue going unresolved only to resurface with other patients.

It has been difficult for Penny at times, working on a teaching unit, seeing residents come through who know less than she does, but whose orders she is required to follow. Some, of course, are really nice. They know they're new. They ask questions. They seek advice. They learn to work as a team. They're not all jerks. Those who are make up for it, though. She blames their education for that and the medical profession in general. Look at the malpractice crisis that's going on. It's been shown that many of the cases involve the same people, again and again. But the medical profession is so entrenched in protecting its own from anyone outside that they do so even when it harms the majority of their own people.

Penny sees it with residents who screw up, like Dick, who

really is the worst that residency has to offer. Sure, they may get counseled or whatever, but once they're in the medical club, the system buffers them and pushes them through. It's like pushing a kid who can't read or write through grade school.

When the community meeting gets under way, Pam's presence is of little concern to the group as a whole. She has a few staunch advocates who sarcastically insist she is being treated so badly that she might as well be muzzled and put on a leash. Her psychiatrist tries twice, unsuccessfully, to mold the group into giving Pam a chance. It's a clear instance of staff splitting, pitting one group against another. Debbie and Rose exchange glances, knowing they'll have to discuss this in their later meeting. It's the kind of behavior they will have to confront at the staff team meeting.

Debbie believes that psych draws people who are looking for help—not just in nursing, but each of the disciplines: psychiatry, social work, art, music, and movement therapies. She thinks this is particularly true of staff drawn to large, conservative private institutions like this one, which emphasizes long-term, introspective therapy. Looking at the people who pass through here, she no doubt sees some of the brightest lights that exist, but many of them are substantially troubled individuals.

She is very clear about her own decision to enter psych. She wanted to know more about herself. She grew up in a household brimming with hidden agendas that needed attending to one way or another. She didn't realize it at the time, but as she began learning about family dynamics in school, lights started going on inside—"Oh, yeah, I recognize that!"

What concerns most of the patients at the meeting is the behavior of a male patient who attempted to burn one of the nurses yesterday. Donna had wanted to do a nursing care plan with Kevin, a twenty-four-year-old schizophrenic who had been getting increasingly psychotic during the last week. He was a voluntary patient who had the right to refuse medications. His mood swings had become more pronounced with brief outbursts of irrational rage, but he hadn't done anything that would allow his psychiatrist to start involuntary commitment proceedings. The staff all agreed that by not demanding to sign out of the hospital, he was nonverbally communicating his need for help, "on some level."

Many of the other patients had complained about him throughout the week, growing apprehensive as he became more uncommunicative and paced the halls, mumbling curses and giggling to himself. The behavior wasn't all that unusual on the unit, but Kevin was a big guy. Though more fat than muscle, he was intimidating.

Donna had taken him to a quiet part of the hall to talk. They sat on a couch, and he asked her for a cigarette. Normally, in order to maintain therapeutic boundaries, the custom is that staff don't give their own things to patients. But, being a fellow smoker, Donna could relate to his request.

They hadn't been talking more than a few minutes, nothing very significant, "So how're things going for you?" types of questions, when Kevin tried to burn her arm with the cigarette.

"His therapist can read whatever he likes into that," Donna had said to Penny during report yesterday. "But it was scary, and I beat it out of there for help. It was okay afterward, though. He was downright docile. He went into seclusion without any problem. We didn't even have to do an 'All call.' "

Because Kevin refused to attend the meeting, other patients felt free to express their anger at him and their fear. Penny assured them it was a single incident, that he'd been compliant afterward, that he had been placed on arson precautions, meaning he could only have cigarettes if a staff member was with him, and that the staff would continue to do whatever was possible to protect every person on the unit.

"Protect us," an adolescent scoffs. "You can't even get us all down to breakfast."

Laughter erupts around the circle until the depressed bonds trader Debbie spoke with earlier breaks in sarcastically, "Do you call having someone here with AIDS protecting us?"

Harry shifts uncomfortably in his seat, his face flushed, eyes to the floor. Ken, beside him, well within arm's reach, is poised for action. However, a chorus of voices chastise the speaker, a verbal skirmish about right to know versus right to privacy ensuing.

An uneasy silence follows, stretching throughout the remainder of the meeting. The staff tries several avenues of contact without success. When Debbie directly mentions Adelle Y., the woman who had committed suicide, a flurry of seat changing and throat clearing spreads about the circle. One woman bursts out in tears.

"Nice going!" a manic-depressive man hisses.

"It's all right to cry," the attending psychiatrist assures everyone.

Penny is working with two patients now who she believes will commit suicide. They are depressed over truly tragic situations in their lives. One woman was pinned in a car crash, unable to reach her daughter, who bled to death in the backseat. The other is a young man who was sexually abused and physically battered by his father for years on end. When they talk about suicide, she believes them, a gut feeling.

Sometimes Penny will party pretty hard as a means of coping. Some days she deals with it by playing a role, the role of *the nurse*. What would the nurse do in a case like this? It's time for the nurse to pour medications.

"Sometimes I have to remind myself why I became a nurse in the first place. It's not a bad reason. I truly wanted to help people."

She has been trying to exercise more. That helps. It's better than drinking. What works the best—say when she's been working a protracted string of evenings—is to set her alarm and force herself up to go work out. Then she has some productive time during the day before going in to face it again, and at night she doesn't feel as much like going out for drinks, partying, and sleeping the next day away. Still, it's hard to break bad habits.

After community meeting, Suzanne, as charge nurse, breaks seclusion with two techs, Ken and Katy. Rose listens on the microphone. The plan Suzanne proposes to Pam is the typical step process for coming out of LDS. The door will remain open for an hour, but Pam is to remain inside, demonstrating her ability to control her impulsiveness. She agrees, also agreeing to remain "zoned" to the community room, where she can be easily observed once out of seclusion. But she continues to refuse to disclose the razor's location.

"Pam," Suzanne informs her, "we're really concerned that another patient might find it and harm themselves."

Suzanne has a generally good rapport with Pam, being her primary nurse.

"Oh, Suzanne—pa-lease!" Pam drawls. "Guilt? You're gonna try guilt? With me?"

"It was worth a try," Suzanne admits, and both laugh.

Forty percent of Debbie's time is spent on formal staff teaching. She orients new employees to the hospital, supplying them with basic psychological concepts, such as how to tell their own and the patient's superegos apart, or recognize transference and counter-transference. She teaches aggression management techniques, such as how to safely work seclusion scenes. She'll do in-service work, usually focused around particular problems identified by the staff or head nurses. It's her contribution to comb the literature and pull together a presentation.

The other 60 percent is clinical and is as varied as the floors are. On one floor, she has been involved in a series of role-playing therapies with a few patients. She was brought in at the request of a psychiatrist who was having difficulty connecting with a regressed patient who hated her mother. Debbie and the doctor worked out the focus of the therapy, and she went to work. The results were so positive that she was tapped to work with a few other patients.

Recently, it has been necessary to have numerous interdisciplinary meetings around the issue of the tremendous staff turnover, with resulting conflicts about "who's-in-control?" issues, themes of powerlessness over decision making and a lot of finger pointing. The staff has really been caught in the mud. Debbie came in at Rose's request to support nursing—which was getting rained on mightily by everybody else.

Debbie sympathizes with Rose's problems, considering the head nurse position the most stressful in the hospital, being too pivotal with too many demands. No other team member has responsibility for thirty-six individuals—twenty patients and a staff of sixteen: RNs, psych techs, and a unit clerk—any one of whom her ADN (assistant director of nursing) might inquire about at any time. And she had damn well better know the answer or have the information available shortly. Head nurses are always in a catch-up mode, always responding to people asking, "Why didn't you?" "How could you?" "I needed it yesterday!"

Debbie was a head nurse here from 1975 to 1984. It was a long-term unit, mostly schizophrenic and character-disorder patients. To a large extent, she learned to be a head nurse by recalling what *not* to do, by doing the opposite of how she had been treated as a staff nurse. When she started in the field, in a Catholic hospital, nurses were expected to stand when a nun walked into a room. Coming from a Quaker background, she didn't know the difference between nuns and priests or the associated rituals, and was constantly getting gigged for breaching some shrouded ground rule. As head nurse, she made a point of introducing new people to as many unspoken norms as she could articulate.

Turnover problems happen at times for no discernable reason and can have a devastating impact on a unit. In one eighteen-month span while a head nurse herself, Debbie went through twenty-six staff members for twelve positions. It was awful.

There was always somebody in orientation, always someone struggling to get a foothold, always somebody who had an evaluation due. It was not unusual to get a staff transfer from another hall—an involuntary transfer, someone who'd been told, "Look, they need help up on that unit and it's *you* . . ."—about which Debbie was given very little choice. If it was someone who knew the system, it was fine, but usually they were those with the least seniority, often requiring orientation from scratch. Conversely, during periods of staff stability, she lost people being pulled to other floors needing help.

As long as there was a core of people who were well grounded—say, a third of the staff—Debbie felt she could manage. There were one RN and two psych techs in particular who had been with her for a couple of years—strong, reliable people. She got to the point where if the unit lost two or three staff members within a short period—like in the summer, when everybody went to find themselves going cross-country or to Europe—as long as the core remained, she could tolerate the lack of confidence and competence in the rest.

Then, within two days of one another, both techs resigned. That ripped it. Debbie was as burned out as she had ever been. Charbroiled, deep fat fried. There were no boundaries, no walls. Work spilled over into her personal life and vice versa. Everything got blurry. It was a time of free-floating discontent. She was angry at the nursing administration, furious with the doctors, the social worker, and the activity therapists, and royally pissed off at the service chief. Everyone was just so goddamn incompetent. There was a medical student she could have murdered. And she was so very, very tired. No matter what she did, it wasn't enough.

"I guess I'm supposed to be a good little girl now, right?" Pam yawns, walking to her room with Suzanne. They are about the same size, slender and similar as sisters, Pam's blond hair acquired, Suzanne's brunet from birth.

"That might be refreshing," Suzanne conjectures. "Why not give it a try?"

"Maybe they could take us both down to the ECT room and give us a personality transplant. *Then* tell me how easy it is to be nice."

"Touché." Suzanne feigns a heart stab.

"But I like you too much to wish you were me."

Pam is to be allowed to dress in street clothes before being lounge-confined.

"Can I have my cigarettes, too?"

"I don't see why not."

Pam's room is in disarray, clothing slumped everywhere. She holds up two blouses for inspection.

"Black or white?" she smiles. "This is a test."

"Why, white, of course."

Pam tosses the white blouse over her shoulder, billowing toward the bed.

"How did I know?" Suzanne asks.

"We should go shopping sometime."

When Penny is halfway back to the hall to continue an NCP conference with a patient, the doorbell sounds again. Because it is a locked unit, all visitors and patients need to ring and wait while a staff person comes to evaluate their entry. It is a nursing staff function, keeping the unit running. Penny returns to unlock the door. It is a patient she just let out.

"Sorry," the girl says. "Forgot my sunglasses. I won't be a sec', I promise."

Ideally, Penny's position entails a lot of patient contact, a lot of counseling-type conversation, while she assesses a patient's health in general. Much time is spent on working with the more regressed, psychotic patients, helping them perform the simplest tasks, such as bathing, dressing, and eating while waiting for the medications to take effect, hoping to build a human bridge of trust between them. It's what drew her to psych. Then there are the co-leading of groups, the participation in activities, the talking to families.

"You do a lot of talking. And, hopefully, some listening. You do a lot of writing, too. Whatever you talk about goes down on paper, in a progress note, in an NCP, on a flow sheet, usually on all three. Rule Number One is always this: If it isn't documented, then it didn't happen."

She enjoys talking with people, understanding the need for connectedness. There's a click that occurs when a patient says something and a light goes on inside, a recognition. Something they may not even know themselves. Something she can verbalize for them. They look at her with that look of "yes"— maybe even saying it, perhaps openly, their own light beaming, perhaps warily, sizing her up for safety—and she feels a bond starting. There's a good feeling that comes from that. Those times, when they happen, are so vital to therapeutic momentum, applying the tissuey layers of trust, gauze upon a burn.

She sees new nurses come in needing to help people, wanting to connect and give. She catches herself modulating her conversations with them, trying not to be too cynical, trying not to burst their bubbles. She sees how much better they feel connecting with somebody, discovering which patients they will work best with.

Adele is the first suicide Penny has had to deal with. She'd come in extremely depressed, feeling like nothing, no one, the zero after the decimal point. But she'd rallied quickly. Several of the staff had premonitions about her. They used to discuss it: "Is she getting *too* well *too* fast?" It is common knowledge that when people have been in deep depression, they are most vulnerable to suicide as they begin to recover, the lid of depressive confusion and lethargy lifting just enough to take action on self-hatred, but not enough to genuinely feel better.

But Adele had made reasonable plans for after discharge, her antidepressants were at the therapeutic level, and things seemed to be going well. There was no way to justify the intuitive dread of the staff. But two weeks after discharge, she was dead.

She was someone Penny felt close to. There was that click of recognition.

"How can you know that about me?" she would ask when Penny hit on things she wanted to say but couldn't. Or things she wanted kept hidden.

   "She didn't know how to express feelings. She was a good person, but she just couldn't see it. If she could just see what I saw. So often people don't see themselves. Maybe none of us do."

Penny misses her—not that she would have kept in touch with her after discharge. But the sense of tragedy lingers. She'll think of her at the strangest times—showering, shaving her legs, just before sleep. Her memory can still touch off tears. She used to tell Penny she wanted to be like her because she would watch Penny walk down the hall with such confidence. She wanted to know how to get that. This was a woman in her sixties. She'd had breast cancer and a mastectomy. She'd beaten it. Talk about ripping your heart out . . .

Suzanne jots down lab results of lithium and antidepressant blood levels for several patients. Hanging up the phone, she finds a student nurse awaiting her attention.

"Excuse me," the student whose name she has forgotten says. "But isn't Kevin still on arson precautions?"

When Suzanne nods, the girl tells her he has been walking up and down the hall with a lit cigarette, dropping ashes at random on the rug, in the wastebaskets, in the water fountain. Suzanne steps to the door. Kevin, his blue jeans slung low beneath his gut, ambles halfway out of the lounge, turns, and wanders back again, smoke rising from his cupped hand.

As Suzanne reaches the lounge, she hears him belch and giggle. An older female patient shakes her head, glares at Suzanne, and returns her attention to her needlepoint.

"Kevin." Suzanne speaks, but he turns away, gazing through the security-screened window. "Kevin, c'mon, you know you're on arson precautions. You need to put out the cigarette. There's an ashtray there. Take a drag and put it out, okay?"

He ignores her, shaking his head almost imperceptibly. Suzanne tries several more times, trying to be as nonthreatening as possible. He finishes the cigarette. Fishing inside his shirt, he extracts another, crosses the lounge to the wall-mounted lighter, and lights it up.

Suzanne returns to the office where Ken is charting vital signs. She tells him what is going on and asks if he will alert the others that she is calling the supervisor for backup to put Kevin in the quiet room. The supervisor arranges to have several male staff members from other units come to Suzanne's hall.

Kevin is seated in a Windsor chair in the corner, chuckling to himself, a curving fingernail of ash growing off the tip of his cigarette, when the staff group approaches. Silence falls over the other patients and two visitors who grow attentive to the scene. Wanting to draw him away from the gaze of the group, Suzanne asks Kevin to accompany her to the nurses' station to discuss this. Again, he ignores her, taking a deep drag, blowing the smoke out toward his cowboy boot sitting atop his knee.

The plan is to have him surrender his cigarettes and take a time-out in the QR. The group of male staff members form a semicircle around him, a "show of force" that, it is hoped, will obviate any violent outbursts.

"Kevin," Suzanne says flatly, "we need for you to give us your cigarette pack. We'll keep it in the office for you. We're worried about you dropping ashes on the floor. Because we're all locked in here, a fire could be a very dangerous thing. We're concerned about your safety and everyone else's."

Kevin remains unresponsive, a doltish, dull distance in his eyes.

"Kevin," Suzanne says soothingly, "we're not trying to hassle you, but we have to think about the safety of everyone here. Can you at least tell me what you think of what I said?''

When he doesn't respond, a tech from another hall reaches out and snatches the cigarette from Kevin's hand, startling everyone; the decision to instigate such action should fall to the charge nurse. Kevin erupts. His boot catches Suzanne in the belly, doubling her over. He lashes out at the other staff members who swarm over him. Within seconds, the overhead intercom is broadcasting the emergency alarm—a whistle code followed by the operator's voice: ''ALL STAFF CALL'' and the location. The routine is to immobilize the violent person facedown on the floor, arms and legs pinned behind his back. It takes several minutes, Kevin snorting and swearing and straining against the bodies atop him.

Other patients and visitors look on in shock. One of the adolescent girls, who has a history of having been sexually abused, clenches her fists, trembling on the periphery of the fray, screaming, ''Stop it! You'll suffocate him! You're killing him! Give him a chance, you bastards!''

Debbie and Rose are out of their snack-bar seats as soon as the hollow whistle sound goes off. They are out the door as the location is announced. They race down the hallway toward the elevator bank. Debbie already has her supervisor's key in hand. It allows her to override the elevator's destination, pulling it to her position. There was a time when she would take the stairs, but she'd like to have some energy left in case she needs to tussle with someone on arrival.

They ascend in silence. Reaching the door, Debbie sees the crowd of bodies outside the seclusion room. They race along the hall, Rose taking the lead. Debbie sees Suzanne, ashenfaced and shaking, seated on a couch, several patients solicitously surrounding her. She can also read the stunned concern on Rose's face.

''Check on Suzanne,'' Debbie says. ''I'll go down here.''

In the seclusion room, someone is still struggling beneath a pile of staff bodies. There are clusters of flying hands pursuing different goals—unlatching Kevin's belt, unbuttoning his shirt, yanking at his boots. Patients need to be disrobed before being restrained.

"Get his boots off first," Ken commands.

Once, at a particularly raucous restraining scene, a staff member's leg was braced and belted before he could tell what was happening.

"Kevin." Penny crouches in a corner near his head. "Listen to me, Kevin. No one is going to hurt you. We are not here to hurt you. If you stop fighting, we can let up on you. . . ."

His thrashing continues. He emits a pained-straining moan as he attempts to dislodge the bodies atop him.

"I'm going to get you some medicine."

"No!"

"Yes, Kevin," Penny asserts. "Yes. Now will you take it by mouth, or do I need to get a needle?"

He curses her, and she spryly avoids the heaving heap of limbs.

In the med room, Penny flips open the Kardex to Kevin's p.r.n. sheet, unlocks the cabinet with the needles and syringes, choosing a three c.c., and snaps the top off a glass ampule of Haldol, a powerful antipsychotic. Realizing she is trembling, she takes a second to steady her hands, then draws up some Ativan for anxiety, some Cogentin for side effects from the Haldol, and returns with all three syringes to seclusion. Kevin has been stripped and a bed brought into the room, his ankles and wrists secured in leather cuffs strapped to the bed frame. He continues to struggle and fume. A towel is held over his mouth to keep his spit from hitting anyone, but his mouth is very dry anyway. These meds will make it dryer.

Penny has learned to deal with psychotic outbursts—the challenge of entering another's rage and soothing it, redirecting it. One part of her will be cringing, thinking, "Holy shit, this can't be happening!" as someone throws a chair, breaks a lamp, threatens fractures and lacerations. But another part seems to disengage and function: "I'm gonna handle this now."

Seclusion and restraining scenes are one of the things psych staff need to get used to dealing with. Locking someone in a room, barren except for a thin mattress on the floor, or tying them to a bed with leathers is often difficult to perceive as "helping." It feels like punishment, certainly for patients and often for new staff, rather than assisting someone to control his or her unruly impulses.

Penny doesn't mind holding someone down in order to give an IM injection or get some nutritional drink down an NG tube. There is a part of her that steps back and doesn't get involved, able to do what is best for the person in the long run rather than feel his or her terror and rage. Plus, it's always done as part of a group. A sort of camaraderie exists because they have helped each other through it, so nobody, not patient nor staff, got hurt.

"I'm so sorry, Suzanne. Oh, God, I'm so sorry," Pam keeps repeating as Rose sits beside Suzanne, arm around her shoulders, insisting she be taken down to the medical office for a checkup.

"I'm okay, really, Rose."

"No, no, you're not. Not until you get checked out. I'm going to have Katy take you down in a wheelchair."

"Rose." Suzanne blanches. "Get a grip. I'd feel stupid. I can walk."

"I will not take any chances with your well-being."

"This is embarrassing."

"I'm so sorry, Suzanne," Pam pleads, tearing up. "Please forgive me."

"Pam," Rose snaps. "What are you talking about?"

"I gave him the cigarettes. Oh, I'm so stupid. Please forgive me, Suzanne?"

"You what?" Rose asks.

"It was just a stupid joke."

Rose reigns in her temper and says, "Pam, please just go have a seat while I take care of this.'' Even with Suzanne hurt, Pam still has to grab center stage. "We'll deal with other things later.''

"Rose, really, I'm okay,'' Suzanne demurs.

"Suzanne, stop acting like a nurse and accept some help.''

"Oh, damn it, I'm so dumb!'' Pam shrieks, storming down the hall. "I could just kill myself!''

Rose looks at Suzanne with a can-you-*believe*-this? expression.

"Go, Rose.'' Suzanne motions. "Go.''

Pam speeds by as Penny exits the seclusion room, Rose in pursuit. Christ, not another one. She lays the empty syringes atop a counter inside the nurses' station, then follows two techs to Pam's room, where Rose has her cornered.

"I think she put something in her shirt.''

"Go to hell, Rose.''

Rose wants to say, You mean I'm not there already?

"I need to check inside your shirt.''

"Lesbo,'' Pam spits.

"If we have to take it off, we will. You know that, Pam.''

Pam sizes them up for a moment and hears others arriving outside. Debbie cracks the door and enters.

"Penny can look, not you.''

"Fine,'' Rose says. "I'll wait outside.''

"And take the goons with you.''

Everyone is keeping a straight face, trying to remain unprovoked. Rose files out with the techs, whispering to Debbie, "We'll be right outside.''

Debbie nods, remaining just inside the doorway. Pam protests until Penny insists her presence is necessary.

Penny pauses a few seconds after the door closes before speaking.

"So, Pam.'' She draws the words out slowly for seriocomic effect. "What's going on?''

Pam cracks a slight smile.

"Just the usual idiocy, I guess, Penny.''

Penny nods sympathetically, although she doesn't much like Pam.

"Well, shall we get this over with?" she asks. When performing tasks she hates, like going through someone's belongings looking for items that might be dangerous or doing a strip search, Penny will usually try to make light of it, tell them she went to nursing school to satisfy an urge to be nosy; that she knew if she became a psych nurse, she could look through people's dirty laundry. "Let's do this scene from *Girls Behind Bars* and then go have a cup of tea."

Pam removes her shirt and does a twirl, showing her there is nothing to see. Penny has her unlatch her bra and hold it away from her body.

"Just shake it," Penny tells her so Pam won't have to take it all the way off.

Pam stares flatly at her.

"I *beg* your pardon," she says, arching an eyebrow.

"I meant the bra."

Then they both start laughing.

"You think Suzanne will be okay?" Pam buttons her blouse, shaking her hair loose from her collar.

"Yeah. She's tough."

"I can't tell you how much I hated to see her get hurt."

"Remind you of your past?"

Pam stops, staring at Penny, who reaches up and gingerly straightens her collar. Pam nods.

"Pam," Penny asks after measuring her a moment. "Where's that razor?"

"I flushed it down the toilet." She shrugs.

"Good. Let's go back up to the lounge now and see Suzanne, okay? Lunch'll be up soon."

On the way out, Debbie holds the door open. As Pam passes through, Debbie gently clasps Penny's elbow and whispers, "Nice work."

8

"The Whole Thing Right There"

The Operating Room

Mavis has had a career-long nightmare that recurs in times of stress. She is alone with her patient in the OR. She has administered a muscle relaxant and paralyzed the patient, taking away his ability to breathe. Inserting a tube into the esophagus, she reaches blindly back for the tubing connector to the anesthesia machine but feels nothing. Turning, she realizes someone has taken away her machine. That's when the terror sweats start. There's nothing she can do but blow down the tube.

Private-hospital operating rooms usually run on schedule. In the university-affiliated hospital in New Mexico where Mavis has practiced as a certified registered nurse anesthetist (CRNA) for more than a decade, this is rarely the case. Each morning, assignments are posted on the board, but by midday that list may have doubled with unplanned surgeries—from the patient reevaluated by his physician during morning rounds to the Lamaze delivery that suddenly needs to be a C-section. ER trauma admissions alone account for approximately a quarter of all OR activity.

Most people don't realize that in the majority of surgical procedures performed throughout the country, the person administering the anesthetic—the person responsible for keeping the patient breathing, monitoring his vital signs, and intervening should anything go wrong—is not a doctor, an anesthesiologist, but a nurse, a nurse anesthetist. This figure rises to 85 percent in rural areas where most anesthesiologists are loathe to locate their practices. CRNAs are also the predominant anesthetists in the military.

Roughly 50 percent of CRNAs are employed by hospitals; the other half split between employment by physicians and being independent contractors. In Mavis's hospital, it is policy to try to keep someone available for contingencies, like ER trauma cases. There is an OR devoted to trauma, no other patients permitted. Sometimes it gets so tight that other procedures must be delayed, but generally the really bad trauma comes at night and on weekends. When trauma cases are absent, there are more mundane needs to be addressed, a float person to step in to sub for coffee, lunch, and bathroom breaks for both CRNAs and anesthesia residents during lengthy surgeries, someone to retrieve extra equipment when needed, and someone who can lend an extra pair of expert hands.

"You can't say to the person next to you, 'Hey, watch my patient, will ya? I wanna go to the bathroom.' You have to have backup. Mostly it's me."

Relieving someone, Mavis enters the OR scrubbed, gloved, gowned, and masked. She checks the digital readouts on the overhead monitor banks—body temperature, blood pressure, heart rate, tidal ventilation, and CO_2 acid-base balance. Blood oxygenation is monitored with a simple finger stick. She reviews the selection of drugs or agents being used, quickly scanning the flow sheet kept going at all times, and gets a quick report from the person she is spelling.

When Mavis came to this hospital, there were only one staff anesthesiologist and a handful of CRNAs. Today, anesthesiology has become a university chair with a burgeoning residency program. CRNAs and anesthesiology residents are scheduled in the OR on a rotating basis. A staff anesthesiologist supervises three ORs at one time, available should complications arise. CRNAs are not restricted by types of cases, performing exactly the same as residents. Heart bypass, neurologic, neonatal, pediatric, obstetrical, and dental cases all pass through their care. Even electroconvulsive (ECT) treatments for psychiatric patients are cared for by them.

The OR is always interesting and often pleasant. Music usually plays while the work proceeds. There are light moments, when for example, nature intrudes amid the high tech: there was a fly in the OR, flitting from surface to surface, shooed from faces and surgical site, uncatchable and unsmashable. It is procedure for the circulating nurse to keep a count of instruments and sponges, a list chalked on a board for double-checking at the end of the operation lest anything be sewn inside the patient. When the fly could not be captured, it was simply added to the list to be accounted for before the incision was closed.

Abrupt, unforeseen changes in a patient's condition are a common occurrence. It is a challenge Mavis thrives on, proud of her ability to diagnose a problem and take steps to correct it, and CRNAs are able to correct problems without asking anyone's permission. Mavis can perform invasive procedures and place arterial or central monitoring lines, evaluating them herself. She can float a Swan-Ganz catheter directly into the circulatory system to assess exact heart functioning status if she thinks it is needed. She can perform whatever anesthetic blocks she is capable of—spinals, epidurals, regional blocks.

Mavis prefers a conservative approach, looking disdainfully on those who want to jump right into potent medications as soon as the blood pressure drops. It's possible to try fluid increases or other measures before whipping out a syringe of epinephrine.

Anesthetists wear an earpiece with tubing on it that fits into an esophageal stethoscope down the throat with which they can listen to the heartbeat and lung movements. When oxygenation starts falling, something bad is happening. The tone of the machine drops with the oxygenation.

"You can hear it, especially with a child, the saturation falling as the coronaries tighten. You're trying to get a tube in to correct whatever is happening, and there is this constant falling sound of absorbing oxygen. When you finally ventilate the patient, you can hear the lung sounds and then the heart—bump, ba-bump.

"It doesn't matter what's happening; if you ventilate and have a good heartbeat, you know you can fix whatever it is. Still, it's very frightening. You can really get into tight spots. Hopefully, you can get out of them."

She may go into a case deciding to use one particular muscle relaxant, only to discover that it drops the blood pressure and that she will have to change to something else. She may want to use one particular agent or narcotic but finds the patient doesn't tolerate it well. That's when she has to intervene, and quickly. There isn't a half hour to ponder it, more like half a minute.

Mavis distinctly remembers the very tiny newborn baby girl admitted for a ventriculoperitoneal (VP) shunt, used to relieve hydrocephalus. The child had multiple congenital problems including nonfunctioning adrenal glands, those small bodies sitting atop the kidneys that produce hormones and are essential for life.

As soon as Mavis intubated her patient, the child's heart stopped. The monitor line went flat, straight across, its neutral hum jarring everyone in the room to do what they could to save her. Perhaps it was the stress of intubation, perhaps it was just her time, but none of the measures employed resuscitated that child.

"I felt very bad, even though I knew it was not my fault and the child would not have lived anyway. The brain stem was not well developed. Still, I felt I lost that child. She came to me alive, kicking her little feet, reaching her little hand out. Twenty minutes later she was dead."

Mavis did her basic nursing training in the West Indies, a very British-type program. It took four years, with a diploma awarded upon completion. Afterward, it was customary for graduates to go into midwifery, requiring another year of training. Mavis didn't like midwifery, though, and got out almost immediately, preferring a variety of experiences—medical and surgical, pediatrics and clinics. Even a stint in physiotherapy.

Leaving the islands in the late fifties, she came to New York City, where she would remain for eighteen years before moving to the Southwest. At that time, individuals seeking nursing licensure were evaluated upon what training they had already received. Deficiencies were dealt with through remediation—in her case, psychiatry, not taught in the islands—and testing. New York State then bestowed a "license by endorsement," recognized only by the state, without reciprocity elsewhere.

She worked a surgical ward, a medical floor, the recovery room, and the OR as a scrub nurse before deciding upon anesthesia. At that time, in the mid-sixties, all that was required for acceptance into anesthesia school was an RN license. Training lasted twenty-six months at the Harlem Hospital of Medicine. After anesthesia school, she decided she wanted to have a "license by exam," so that she might have reciprocity anywhere. She sat for the state boards in the early seventies.

Today, most nurse anesthetist programs are at the master's level, taking anywhere from two to three years, depending upon thesis-writing time or the individual student's scientific background.

"I had a very interesting life, professionally. I finished nursing and anesthesia and still didn't have a college degree. Since everybody has at least a bachelor's degree in nursing these days, I said to myself, 'You need a college degree.' So I went back to college. I went into health education also and took a master's degree in that as well, which I completed in Albuquerque in '82."

Anesthesia is clearly the area of practice Mavis most enjoys. The autonomy of the position allows her to do things that no other nursing speciality ever did, truly making diagnoses that make a difference. Variety exists in both illness and individual. Even if she does hysterectomies every day, each patient is a little different, responding uniquely. That's exciting, fueling her interest.

Treatment choices, too, are different: one patient choosing to use an epidural or a spinal, another to be put to sleep. Being able to discuss choices with patients—letting them know they don't have to go to sleep if they don't want to—adds the human element to this highly technical field. Some people are scared to go to sleep. Having a choice, as most healthy patients do, helps them feel better.

Mavis will meet with patients for maybe twenty minutes right before surgery, a brief but crucial time, answering questions, explaining what will happen. Even if she saw them the night before, it's best to touch base again just before when anxieties truly begin to spike, when denial and bravado crumble. She tries to let them get to know her quickly. She is a robust woman who exudes compassion, warmth, and confidence. Her voice, retaining its island inflections, is smooth and calming. Being as straightforward as she can, she wants them to know she can be trusted to be there for them no matter what happens.

"I'm gonna be right there with you the whole time. We're gonna do all these different things to make sure you're comfortable. And we'll do everything we can to make sure you come through this okay."

She enjoys her ability to bring reassurance to patients. Even though the risk of death under anesthesia is slim, it is always there. Usually her presence alone is calming enough. If someone goes into surgery in a very nervous state, it can make for a long day with blood pressure rollercoasting, adrenaline splashing through the system, the whole spectrum of somatic anxiety at play. If she can foresee these problems for such individuals, Mavis will sedate them before they go into the OR. She calls it "slowing them down." Some patients don't remember the OR at all.

The American Association of Nurse Anesthetists was founded in 1931. Today its membership numbers more than 23,000 CRNAs, a 98 percent representation rate, the highest for any nursing speciality organization. Membership dues are $300 annually. One of its functions has been to act in an advisory capacity when CRNAs believe they are being discriminated against by the medical community. Arguments continue to float back and forth between CRNAs and the medical community, often centering around credentialing and cost-effectiveness.

Roughly twenty million procedures requiring anesthesia are performed each year in the U.S., the cost hovering somewhere in the vicinity of $3 billion. The anesthesiology-residency program lasts for four years. As with all medical specialities, board certification is voluntary, but becoming the norm. It is one of the fastest-growing medical specialities, with some of the highest compensation in medicine. American Medical Association figures in 1989 place the average salary at $185,800.

To be a certified registered nurse anesthetist requires a baccalaureate degree in a science-related field, usually a BSN, and a year of critical care nursing prior to entry. Programs range from twenty-four to thirty-six months with a minimum of 375 didactic hours—pathophysiology, chemistry, physics, pharmacology, etc.—and 800 hours of anesthesia required for completion. As of June of 1989, there were ninety-four programs recognized by the Council on Accreditation of Nurse Anesthetists. In 1990, a government survey estimated a shortage of six thousand to seven thousand certified registered nurse anesthetists.

Unlike anesthesiology, passing a national certification exam is mandatory before a license to practice is awarded. Forty hours of continuing education units (CEUs) are also needed every two years for recertification. It's necessary for Mavis to keep her RN and CRNA licenses up-to-date, both the state nursing board and the AANA requiring proof of the other's validity.

In 1989, a University of Texas survey placed the average CRNA salary in the mid-$50,000 range. According to AANA figures, this can increase into the low $100,000s for those who own their own businesses. Liability rates are also impressive. When Mavis left anesthesia school in the mid-sixties, she paid fifty-two dollars for three years of coverage. Today, the average CRNA pays about $6,000 each year. It can be double or triple that amount, depending upon where the practice is located. A 1986 congressional bill made anesthetists the first nursing speciality to receive direct reimbursement under Medicare's prospective payment system. A 1985 Health Care Finance Administration study targeted the CRNA bill at $160 million.

CRNAs have been documented in function since 1877. Today, it is legal for CRNAs to practice as long as a physician is present. Any MD will suffice. It does not have to be an anesthesiologist— something anesthesiologists would like to change. It is an important distinction because many anesthetists practice in remote areas where there are no anesthesiologists. Still, anesthesiologists continue attempts to curtail CRNAs in both civilian and military arenas.

Certainly, the aspect of her job that Mavis least appreciates is her occasional collisions with physicians, having them put her down because she is not a doctor. There are the subtle power plays, such as the doctor's saying: "Don't start anything until I get there," a way of letting her know who's in charge. Half the time on busy days the doctor will be called away to something else before he can get there, and she'll proceed with the case anyway.

There are times when the physician will insist that she do something his way instead of the way she planned, such as using a certain drug for induction, based purely on preference and not on any demonstrable superiority. She has never had to sit with a patient and do something she is totally uncomfortable doing, something she felt was dangerous to the patient based upon the patient's history or illness. Nor would she. There is always the privilege of withdrawing from the case if there is something with which she disagrees.

"There are those attitudes that say, 'I'm the doc . . . !' I know that; I don't have to be reminded of that. Maybe he has to remind himself, but that's neither here nor there. Believe me, I don't want to be in their place. I'm a nurse and that's fine. I'm happy to be a nurse. I don't feel that makes me less than anybody else. I know I do an equally important job as the doctor's.

"Other than that, it's a wonderful profession."

Ethical dilemmas of life-and-death decisions are a common refrain in high-tech areas. Organ harvesting is one of Mavis's strangest duties, keeping bodies functioning until the kidney, heart, or some other part can be removed. Pulmonary edema, bronchial clogging, and decreased blood flow to organs must be avoided, electrolyte balance and maximum oxygen saturation maintained. Regular arterial-blood gas checks, suctioning, cadaver positional changes, and blood-product infusions are all employed.

Mavis knows they are being kept alive artificially when they come to her. They have to be declared dead beforehand. Still, they have a good blood pressure that she maintains with the appropriate drugs; their hearts are beating, vital signs normal. Then the kidneys come out and the heart comes out, lung, bone or ear tissue, and corneas. Then Mavis turns everything off, and they die. It feels eerie. In the heart it feels eerie, while the head knows it's right.

There are also the patients who are kept alive, but not without a cost. Mavis has seen someone with a transected aorta quickly placed on the heart-lung machine, the aorta clamped for mending. But, in the meantime, kidney function was being lost and other damage sustained. She has seen the ones kept alive when they should have died, lingering on machines like vegetative mass. She deals with it by treading the technical path, knowing she can only do the best she knows how. Plus, there have been those few patients—enough to keep her going—who she thought should be allowed to die, but who later recovered to be discharged and walked out the door.

The longest operation Mavis ever participated in was a craniotomy that lasted fifteen hours. The patient had a brain tumor. She had a seizure that day and was brought into the hospital. At that time, there were no CAT scans, so a pneumoencephalogram was done. This is a contrast study allowing for visualization of brain lesions. For the first two or three hours, all they did was X rays, pinpointing the problem. It was difficult because the patient was placed in a chair and spun around quickly in order to get all views. Mavis had to remain with her throughout, trying to keep her stable, literally hands-on stable, while checking for ill effects.

When the tumor was found, everyone recognized the need to catch it immediately. Any postponement and the patient would have permanent damage. She was already beginning to have symptoms of the tumor's expansion—headache, vomiting, and visual field disturbances.

Surgery lasted for twelve hours. This was back in the sixties. Ventilators were just becoming a part of the anesthetists' armamentaria. The one Mavis had access to broke that day, and she had to ventilate by hand. Making matters worse was having the surgical point located in the brain. When the brain is swollen, only hyperventilation with 100 percent oxygen will make it constrict. It was necessary to hyperventilate the patient throughout the procedure.

"I couldn't use my arm the next day. But, I'll tell you, when I went to the recovery room, it was worth it all. She was awake and spoke to me. That was the whole thing right there."

9

"This Isn't K Mart"

Recovery Room

Dan is the night-shift, OR-recovery-room nurse in a large North Carolina county hospital. He handles whatever comes out of the OR on the night shift, from kids swallowing hairpins to major trauma like stabbings or motorcycle accidents. The OR/recovery team commits to a narrow focus: get that patient off the OR table alive, get them through post-anesthesia, and return their physiology to a functioning level.

Dan is the only RN—sometimes with an aide, sometimes alone—assigned to the recovery room. If the patient is headed to the ICU, he follows him or her one-on-one. Same for children. With someone headed for a med-surg floor, an appendix or uncomplicated C-section, he'll do two cases alone. Any more than three and he calls for backup.

He tries to tell the OR crew ahead of time if he thinks he'll need help. But patients coming out of anesthesia are always unknown entities. Confusion and nausea are common, lending recovery part of its nickname—"vitals and vomit." Patients sometimes wake up swinging, trying to take his head off. One guy—one *big* guy—confused and furious, flat out extubated himself. He wanted that damn tube out and started yanking it out. It happened so quickly, Dan found himself stretched across the patient, unable to reach the phone two feet away, while the guy was trying to pound him half to death. Luckily, no lasting damage was done to either of them.

Dan has had occasion to call for assistance—to fetch an amp of Lidocaine, for emergency treatment of ventricular arrhythmia, or an antihypertensive such as Apresoline—only to find that the OR staff was out of earshot, setting up rooms for the next cut, leaving him in crunch situations where he had to leave his patient's side; not far away, but farther than he would like.

Staffing shortage is an ongoing debate with administration. Each time there is an incident, Dan sits down with his supervisor and the OR director to review the situation. The standards of the Association of Recovery Room Nurses state that a nurse should never be left alone in a recovery room. There should always be at least an aide present, someone to call for STAT help should the nurse be engaged in resuscitation. His supervisor has told him that both she and the OR director have gone to administration with the problem and been told pointedly that no new night-shift staff will be added, budgetary considerations overriding objections.

"I don't know what goes through administrators' minds. I'm talking about lives, and they're talking about money. My opinion is that they're such businesspeople today, these MBAs running hospitals, businesspeople making medical decisions. They run numbers on nurse/patient ratios into a computer and make decisions based on a budget as to how many nurses it's going to take to give safe care.

"They know they're insured. They've got malpractice insurance if something goes wrong. I really believe they look at the odds, the percentage chance of something going wrong, and then the chance of being sued if it does, instead of covering it so that you get it 100 percent right. I've been real lucky so far, and I don't want that to change."

Dan carries his own malpractice insurance, his most recent premium tripled for six-months' coverage. It angered him enough to change companies, but his disgruntlement lessened after he talked with the nurses over in labor and delivery. They had been paying $56.00 yearly when it jumped up over $500 in a single hike. Many of those nurses are talking about leaving that area of work.

Dan spends so much time in the recovery room that it feels like a second home. He'll judiciously bend rules on occasion—"NO VISITORS PERMITTED IN THE RECOVERY AREA"—to accommodate families, particularly parents. If he knows there are anxious family members waiting outside, pacing off the dead-weight hours of a surgical procedure—and that the surgeon may or may not speak to them when it's over—Dan will bring them back into the lounge, where a pot of coffee is always brewing and music is playing, and let them ask their questions, express their guilt or dismay, and try to demystify the surroundings. Simply seeing where their family member will be spending the next few hours can go a long way toward alleviating apprehension.

He believes in bringing a lot of color into the hospital, making it more user-friendly. He grows roses and will sometimes sneak some in to leave on desks anonymously. He plays a hammer dulcimer in local bars and coffeehouses, and often brings it in to play for patients. Many of the patients are children, so he's learned to juggle. The kids wake up after surgery crying, terrified, wanting their moms, unsoothed by word or gesture. But pull out three beanbags, start juggling and humming, and suddenly the climate changes, they are engaged in more than their fear.

Autonomy is Dan's principle motivation for working the graveyard shift, the ability to express some creativity, to have some flexibility of function. After almost ten years in the field, most of it in critical care areas, he enjoys using his skills. Med-surg floor work just didn't suit him: walking around assessing breath and bowel sounds, checking intake and output, keeping an eye on people, doing casual chitchat assessments: "How ya feeling today, Mrs. So-n-so?"

Dan likes to jump into a patient, find out what's going on

inside: what his PA (pulmonary artery) pressure is doing (a measure of left heart function, indicating fluid administration), what his CVP (central venous pressure; measures stress capacity of the circulatory system) and cardiac output say. At any given time, he may be monitoring Swan-Ganz catheters and arterial lines inserted to assess a patient's circulatory and cardiopulmonary stability, deciding when to draw labs for a pH-balance reading, clotting factors, a platelet count, or blood gases or whatever is needed to stabilize that patient before moving him or her along in the chain of recovery.

When he first came to work here, Dan went into the surgical ICU, open-heart recovery, hoping to gain specialized knowledge. As a new nurse, on his third day in a hospital in Ohio, he was dragged into the supervisor's office by the charge nurse. She wanted to establish her ground, make sure he knew who was boss. It was an incident where they had disagreed on something. It came down to her asserting her authority, and mightily. For a scorching half hour, she humiliated him with her superior knowledge.

Moving to North Carolina, Dan went into SICU. It was an aggressive environment where he had to know his stuff to develop a more assertive personality. The staff were barracudas, just eating each other alive. A very competitive, back-stabbing environment. He stuck it out for a year and a half, getting to be a primary nurse for open-heart patients, getting to be as good as any of them, determined that no one ever again could drag him into an office and pummel him with data.

To this day, Dan is certain the incident with his old charge nurse was based upon sexual discrimination, being a male in a female profession. Some of the nurses he later became friends with confessed, "When we heard a man was coming in, there was panic. Everybody was saying, 'He's gonna try and take over!' "

Many female nurses agree that there are sex-specific differences in the treatment of male and female nurses. Kathleen believes that for the most part men are treated with blanket respect where women are treated dismissively or even with hostility. She has witnessed male nurses remain unscathed in situations where a female is reprimanded. She once overheard her head nurse reinforcing the value of paperwork to a man she works with, and he responded, "Oh, that's such a buncha bullshit."

"Now, if I'd ever let the bull-word slip out of my mouth to her, I'd get written up or taken to the director of nursing's office in a flash. There was a female nurse who lost her temper with another employee and said the F-phrase and was docked a day's pay."

Physicians, too, treat male nurses better. If a nurse does something the doctor thinks is a real bozo move, they'll approach a male nurse and say, "Hey, listen, buddy, I think there's a better way to do that. Lemme show you how I learned it in med school." Let a female nurse do the same thing, and they'll come up with a paternal attitude, put a hand on her shoulder, and say, "Hey, honey, let me show you where you screwed up."

Kathleen has witnessed patients treat male nurses deferentially because they think they're doctors. In one instance, she entered a patient's room to help the guy off a bedpan. He was mad because he sat there too long and not a bit bashful about letting her know it.

Asking "Well, sir, who put you on the bedpan?," she heard the man reply, "That doctor did," and say it as if he was so nice to do so in the first place. Then, after clarifying the identity of his nurse for him, the guy started making excuses for him. "Oh, well, I guess he's busy or something."

"He starts out mad at me, even though I'm not his nurse, and he knows I'm not his nurse, but he feels he's got a right to be angry. He doesn't mind taking it out on a woman but doesn't want to confront a man."

In Doris's dual-facility hospital, separate incidents occurred that reeked of preferential treatment for males. In the first, a male physician and a female nurse were discovered having sex on the premises. The nurse was summarily dismissed, while the doctor met with no punitive response. At first, this was interpreted as reflective of the manner in which each profession has traditionally dealt with transgressions—nursing with prompt vindictiveness, and medicine by ignoring the problem.

Then, a year later, in the sister institution, a similar situation was uncovered, only this time it was a female nursing supervisor and a male staff nurse. The supervisor was fired, but the staff nurse remained employed until leaving of his own accord. The argument was made that she, being the supervisor, bore the greater responsibility—and besides *he* was on his break. Still, most believed it revealed a male bias among the administrators making the decision.

Maureen has seen the other side as well, beginning in nursing school when a male student in her rotation was discriminated against by being prohibited from performing certain clinical functions, like inserting Foley catheters in women. One day he was making light of it, like, "Oh, big deal, right?" when she took him to task, saying, "Michael, if I were you, I'd be insulted. You have a right to learn these things. Your money's just as good as any female student's. When you go to a hospital for employment and have to do that, you will not have had the experience, because they excluded you. That's unjust, and you should be outraged."

"We haven't gotten over this sex issue in nursing. They add connotations to nursing functions involving the opposite sex. Now, I'm all for the privacy thing, like if there's some young guy who thinks he's a stud and doesn't want me inserting a catheter, hey, I say fine! if there's somebody else to do it. Well, let's face it, there's not always a male nurse available. Conversely, women have to accept the role of the male nurse. They accept doctors sticking their fingers here, there, and everywhere. Not to mention medical students. So why not a man who's a nurse? Why pretend it's a sex issue?''

Being a male and a nurse, Dan gets to experience some of the worshipful attitude that patients lavish upon physicians, hinging on each utterance as if it were Holy Writ. Patients get a look in their eyes that has equal parts of fear and hope. It's very deferential, as if Dan's got the news from the front lines, as if he can take the terror out of their hearts. It can really inflate the ego. It's very seductive.

Whenever he works with residents right out of medical school, Dan always warns them about that trap and has a lot of respect for the ones who can keep their egos in perspective. There are some terrific doctors Dan regards as having very high character because they haven't let the ''doctor'' name tag change the person they are. That can take an incredibly strong person.

Then there are some who get off on the doctor/God concept who treat nurses very poorly. A good nurse with some experience can take them down quickly, let them know, ''We can help you, or we can make your job very difficult.'' All it takes is for the doctor to write an order like, ''Call doctor if temperature is above 101.'' When that temperature hits 101.1, and it's the middle of the night—and if the nurse is a nitwit or playing paybacks with a doctor who's a jerk—then sure, call. The nurse is already awake. If the doctor wants to give out hard ways to go, then the going gets hard.

''Hey, *you* wrote the order.''

All in all, Dan has a good working relationship with doctors. They tend to approach problems in the same way, to be more task-resolution oriented, to share a team consciousness: if everybody carries out their little job, we can move the ball down the field. He is the first to admit that doctors treat the female nurses a little less respectfully than they treat him, coming to talk to him before approaching them about a patient. He is unsure if that's all a male-to-male thing or is due to the reputation he has acquired for being aggressive in the care of his patients.

Sometimes he'll be cruising around the units on a slow night, and a female nurse will ask him if she should wake up the doctor when the doctor didn't order something correctly, when there are no parameters written, or the dosage is questionable.

"I guess you'll have to. If he didn't cover it correctly. That's why he makes the big bucks, so you can call him at three in the morning and get it corrected."

"But the last time I woke him up, he yelled at me."

Dan isn't certain but thinks such timidity is the reason some of the doctors will seek him out before talking with the female nurses.

His most common conflict with other nurses happens around admissions. Floor nurses hate to get admissions in the middle of the night. There are always a dozen reasons that never make sense—it's too late in the shift, and we don't want to dump it on the next shift; it's too early in the shift, and we haven't organized ourselves yet. They'll cop an attitude at times, as if this is something he is doing to screw up their shift.

"An ad*mission*? Christ! How are we supposed to handle that? What, are you punching them out like widgets up there?"

He doesn't know what they think is going to happen on nights. It's not like it isn't their regular shift. Nursing is the twenty-four-hour profession. An admission's an admission; nobody likes'm, but it's what pays the rent.

The only time he ever gets his supervisor involved in a problem between himself and another staff nurse is with floor nurses around admissions from recovery. When the OR is busy, patients need to be processed. He usually deals with the more overtly hostile confrontations by writing up an incident description and giving it to his supervisor. "This is how I saw what happened. If she goes to her supervisor and makes an issue of it, here's my documentation. If not, then let's just forget it. It's not worth making a fuss."

He's sorry to be the one bringing them all the time, but that's how the system runs.

* * *

Dan's surgical ICU experience was intensely challenging and rewarding, supplying him with a wealth of learning that he has been able to draw on since. Patients arrived with three or four pages of orders, preprinted with parameters filled in by the physical for the particular patient—"keep PCO_2 (carbon dioxide tension; an indication of respiratory status) between X and Y," . . . "Wean at this time, going down by X-amount," etc.— covering just about every contingency. A lot of leeway existed within those parameters for independent judgments, which Dan enjoyed immensely.

Patients stayed a day or two, remaining longer only when infections developed. Then they were sequestered in corner rooms, with drab green blinds over the windows, and received massive care. Reverse isolation techniques were commonly employed: gowning, gloving, and masking each time anyone had contact with the patient to protect the patient from infection. And they hung around for weeks on end. Whenever Dan was assigned to a corner room, he knew he'd bad-mouthed *some-body* he shouldn't have.

With the heart-bypass patients, Dan was dealing with only a half dozen surgeons. He got to know the treatment biases of each one, enabling him to act accordingly when questions arose. It was good for the surgeons, not having to be called in the middle of the night, and good for the patient because problems were dispatched speedily.

The recovery room is different in that there are so many types of surgeons, especially with surgical residents changing every six months. Usually an open-heart patient comes into recovery in the late afternoon. By the next morning, he is extubated and moved elsewhere. One team of surgeons will have that patient to the floor in one day. The other team, who do the second-most surgeries, will have them to the floor in two days. Those teams are great to work with.

Then there's another surgeon. Many of his patients never even get to the floor. He'll do five and six vessel bypasses where the others do only three. He'll pick up the patients the other two teams would tell, "We really think you ought to live your life out to the fullest, enjoy the time you have left and, oh, yes— make out a will." Because this guy will take whatever anybody else refuses, his average of success isn't very high.

"I've got some ethical problems with that in my own mind, but as to the nursing care that comes out of my hands, I give a hundred percent no matter who or what they are. That's what I'm paid to do. Later on, it'll piss me off that this guy did the surgery. He doesn't have a practice that's exactly flourishing, so he has to haunt the halls of nursing homes, pulling people out to do bowel surgery in the middle of the night. Then he gets the government's money. I had to recover a ninety-nine-year-old woman. A nursing-home patient, bedridden. There's something real wrong there."

Many of the elderly, indigent folks from nursing homes have no one to protect their interests. Dan has discussed it with his supervisor. Everybody is aware of what goes on. As far as administration is concerned, they fall back on the tactic "Who are we to decide?"

Dan feels they're ignoring the responsibility to make difficult decisions, like they do in England. Take dialysis patients: in America, the government pays several billion dollars each year for dialysis patients. In England, after age fifty-five, patients have to pay for it themselves. Americans tend to believe that if the technology exists, then everybody should use it, including the bedridden to whom it can't give back a decent quality of life. A full one-third of the health care dollar is spent on people in their last year of life.

Health care rationing is a topic no one wants to mention, as if it didn't already exist, squeezing millions off Medicaid. Millions of working poor are caught in the vise of making too much to qualify for public health assistance but not enough to afford their own coverage. Treating a trauma patient can easily cost $10,000, a heart transplant $100,000. Houston, with the coun-

"In business, that's okay. But this isn't K Mart. It's not like retail, where overstock is returned if it goes out of fashion. If during the day something like a Foley urine catheter is used up, it won't be replenished until the next morning. When I need one immediately, I have to call the central supply room, file a request form, and wait for some guy to bring it up. It's these nickle-and-dime decisions, motivated by business-minded administrators, that drive me nuts. If someone needs a Foley, he needs a Foley! So what if you have a back stock: *some*body will use that Foley."

When Dan started out here in the ICU, in pre-DRG 1983, it emed he had everything he needed. And on the open-heart nit, where massive revenues were generated for the hospital, ey had anything they wanted. It was "Ask and you shall re- ive." They were loaded. In recovery it's just not that way. covery is a dumping ground, generating no profits, controlled a level outside nursing, and is consistently short-supplied.

"It used to be with nursing that we were a profession dom- nated by another profession. Medicine had dominance over ursing. Now, it's worse. Now, nursing is a profession dom- ated by two professions—the AMA *and* the health business dustry. That's what hospitals have become—industries. And killing the care that's given.

"Patients will tell you, nurses are running around and don't ve time to spend with them. Sure, people want the latest nnology, but they're also scared. They want someone to anize it for them."

he runs out of cases—having direct OR follow-up only 5 percent of the time—Dan readies the room for the day efore floating around the critical care units, helping out atever is needed—running errands, trying to pick up the r wandering down to the ER. The variety keeps it in- . The ER is always good for learning experiences, par-

try's fourth-largest AIDS population—70 percent of v
uninsured—spends $12 million a year on treatment. A
can cost $7,000 per patient per year.

Dan foresees rationing as the major medical battl
1990s. It has already appeared as an issue in several
erendums. Oregon received widespread publicity in 19
state legislature's decision to cease Medicaid funding f
liver, and bone marrow transplants. As elsewhere in s
all comes down to a single word: revenue. It is Dan's b
all administration sees is dollars. He had a conversat
one of the anesthesiologists recently, who told him pre
the same thing. This doctor approached an administr
some of his medical/ethical concerns, and all they cou
answer him in business terms. It was like communica
people from another world.

The hospital used to be a not-for-profit corporation
Dan sounds like a contradiction in terms, but it v
recently by a for-profit health care corporation.
1980s, the number of for-profit hospitals doubled a
count for one-fifth of the nation's 7,000 hospitals. [
has become very state-of-the-art since the takeo
administrator, a physician, was rarely ever seer
jokes about "Casper the CEO." The new one is
a good planner, a good builder. He has acquired
(magnetic resonance imaging machine, an ext
cated, expensive diagnostic device akin to a
shot taken costs approximately $1,000) an
mother/baby unit, adding birthing rooms. He
renovations and cleaned the place up, wal
where. It finally looks like a modern hospi
he has done a great job.

On the other hand, there are times whe
to do the job and there are no supplies be
or somebody wanted to limit the "stock
ally said, "Let's reduce our cash on th
working for us instead of tied up in sup

ticularly when trauma alerts are paged. Unless engaged elsewhere, he'll always stop down to see what's been scraped off the pavement. He'll be seeing most of them anyway. It can be rewarding, following patients through their hospital experiences—from ER to OR to recovery until they stabilize, and then he transfers them out to a unit or a floor—getting a good picture of the overall care.

Talking with other staff nurses, he has found AIDS anxiety everywhere. In the fall of 1991, the *Journal of the American Medical Association* published a nationwide survey revealing that 32 percent of all primary-care physicians do not feel obliged to treat individuals with AIDS. In December 1991, *RN Magazine* published the results of a Public Health Service study that stated that while nurses were more likely to feel themselves at risk for HIV infection than physicians were, they were twice as likely to consider themselves obligated to provide care for HIV-positive patients.

Dan has cared for many AIDS patients. Beyond techniques like gloving up for everyone and masking more than in the past, not much in his practice has changed. Physicians in his hospital are voting in closed sessions on testing all OR patients for AIDS.

> "Of course, nurses don't get a vote. We don't count. I feel I should have the right to know if I'm working on someone who has AIDS, who has any condition that may threaten my life. The hospital thinks they've covered that by issuing us these goggles and gloves and telling us to regard any trauma that comes in off the street as a potential AIDS victim. And I get most of them."

The recovery-room staff has felt particularly dumped on recently. Administration has been remodeling the surgical intensive care unit. They cut down on beds and decided to hold patients overnight in the recovery room—two intensive care patients at a time.

That's fine with Dan as long as it's staffed like an ICU; but they have been staffing it with people who don't have any heart training. People are really on edge. One night, he walked in when there were two patients, one an eighty-year-old and the other in her nineties. He got report on both of them, then assessed them for himself. Next, he refused the assignment.

Both were going down the tubes. With the kinds of surgery they'd had and the tendencies those kinds of patients exhibit at that age, that was a given. One was a bowel surgery. The other was a thoracotomy, a surgical incision of the chest wall. For old people, that's rough. There was barely any leeway in their vital signs. With the diastolic already inching into the mid-nineties on both of them and urine output down, the picture just looked grim.

"You guys may not know it yet, but these two are going down fast, like before the night is out."

The nurse who had given report said, "You're right, Danny. I wouldn't accept this assignment alone either."

She'd had previous CCU experience and stayed to work a double shift. Sure enough, both patients turned bad, requiring split-second interventions to retrieve them.

It was Dan's last day before vacation. He went back in on his first day off to see the director of the OR to tell her that it was wrong even to have asked him to do this assignment. After looking over the whole picture, she agreed.

"Why does it have to fall on me to be the bad guy?" he asked. "To have to come in here and refuse an assignment?"

"You're not looked on as being a bad guy. You're just being a Staff Nurse-II, what you are, who's responsible for making those kinds of decisions."

The major concern in the OR currently is the infection rate, rising since the hospital, in a move to economize, reverted to draping surgical patients with cloths, instead of the disposable paper drapes used previously. Nobody likes the damn cloth things, but they're cheaper because they can be sterilized and reused.

After a few people complained, one of the VPs sent out a

memo inviting staff to "Write down your concerns." The memo had a page attached with lines for people to jot down briefly phrased observations. Instead, about fifty nurses wrote out letters. Some were deferential: "Ah, well, sir, I really don't think this is a very good thing because patients seem to not be doing so well. . . ." Others were scathing, writing things like, "You idiots! Give us back the paper drapes! The infection rate is soaring!"

The VP was piqued that they'd written him en masse. He came up and talked with several of the crews, wanting to know *how* they all knew about the infection-rate rise. Who was saying these things? He wasn't so much concerned about what was going on with the infection rate so much as *who* was spreading this information around.

Dan discussed it with several of the nurses, hearing the same refrain: "Who is this man? We're not stupid—we see patients who had surgery in the last week repeatedly coming back for drainage of an abscess. The doctors talk about it all the time because they're very concerned, too. We don't need a risk-management report to tell us what we know. Administration acts like it's the secret of nuclear fission. God help us if staff members can recognize a trend and deduce the cause! God forbid they'd listen to their professional people who are identifying a problem."

Still, there's been no change: the cloths remain. Again, businesspeople making medical decisions. Dan would like to see the public informed of such trends, believing if it were aired, things would change overnight, what with these PR people being hyperconscious about how they're *perceived* by the community.

Dan has entertained the possibility of leaving nursing, though he denies ever having experienced "burnout."

"What I have experienced is 'pissed off.' I doubt such a thing as 'primary burnout' even exists. There's short staffing from administration; there's not having a strong nursing voice

in policy-making; there's being short-sheeted in supplies because the unit isn't a money-maker for the hospital. Those are
real things.

"But burnout? Burnout is a symptom. Administration always wants to put it on the staff: 'Well, Dan, sounds like
you've burned yourself out.' Everybody has heard that more
than once. It's the perfect evasion—administration can seem
sympathetic and not have to make any real changes. 'We're
gonna give you these how-to-handle-stress courses.' Screw
that—how about more staff so the work won't be so hard?''

What really tipped it for Dan was a recent public-relations
program set up by nursing administration. Titled "You Make
the Difference," it was a series of lectures, self-awareness ex-
ercises, and "psycholinguistic modules" geared toward enhancement of job performance. It was held every day for a week,
four hours at a stretch to accommodate each shift, and all employees were required to attend.

"They have money to spend on this but can't hire a nurse's
aide for the night shift?" It all sounded like new age brainwash-
ing. Everyone Dan spoke to described it differently. When a
NICU nurse inquired about this in the "closure" portion of the
program, she was informed, "The program is structured so that
individuals get out of it what they put into it," as though that
answered anything.

Dan asked the coordinator, "Where does working for constructive change within the environment fall on your little spectrum?"

There wasn't an answer for that. It wasn't in the program.

During the final portion of the program, the CEO came in for
a question-and-answer session. Several in the class were
recovery-room people, just off a shift where one of the heart
patients coded and died. Not in the mood for niceties, they raked
him over the coals.

His discomfort was apparent. He told them he was really

upset that morale was so low but that he couldn't understand the hostility.

"It's not just that we're getting the hearts," he was told. "Or that we aren't getting the differential ICU pay that everybody else is getting. It's that not one single person from upper-level management—not the director of nursing, not the vice president, not you—ever walked into that room and simply said, 'Thank you.' "

"I'll have to think that over," he said.

Two days later, the director of nursing came in, hat in hand, to thank everyone. He'd been reamed out, no doubt. Same for the vice president.

"Sometimes basic stuff like that is all it takes. It's easy. Christ, it's cheap! There are some wonderful things that happen in nursing. There are some great highs you can get out of it. Then there's this flip side. It's like a lotus floating in a cesspool."

10

"Always That Surprise"

Speciality Units

Throughout nursing school, Pat worked nights as a nursing assistant in a nursery. Wanting to build upon acquired skills, she applied for a position in that area after graduation. She was told there were none available, but a position in a combined ICU/CCU was proposed.

"Oh, I'm not ready for *that* yet."

"Don't worry," she was assured. "There will be an RN right there with you until you feel comfortable."

Two weeks later, she was on the night shift along with another new grad and two RNs. Between them, they cared for twelve patients, four of whom were on respirators. There were drug ODs, radical mastectomies, botched abortions, and gunshot wounds. The RNs had precious little time to explain procedures or supervise. This was orientation.

No sooner had Pat and the other new grad passed their boards than the RN in charge called out sick. Another RN, who had no ICU experience, was pulled from labor and delivery. Along with an LPN, they cared for a full house of twelve severely compromised people, including a child in a croup tent and someone immobilized in a Stryker wedge frame.

It was initiation by fire, but they survived and their patients survived. There wasn't time to be scared.

There were a lot of codes on that unit. Hardly a week went

by without one. Sometimes there would be two going on at the same time. In the beginning, other people mostly dealt with it; then Pat began to acquire the skill. Her first experience using cardiac paddles terrified her. Right before shocking the patient, she had watched an intern perform the procedure and the electrical charge arced, blowing the paddles out of his hands. Her fright was palpable as she clutched the handles, hands trembling, thumbs poised above the power discharge buttons, voices calling, "Clear!"

"C'mon, Pat, do it," the resident running the code called. "Let's go."

She did. It didn't arc, and nobody else lit up. And the patient lived.

After being on the unit for a few weeks, she started to realize that codes could be exciting as well as terrifying, the adrenaline rushing, a challenge to be met. Pat's way of dealing with codes, like most who need to, was to mute the reality of the situation by becoming very technical-minded. It helps not to think about what is really going on, what is being experienced on an emotional level.

There was one patient who arrested thirty-seven times on a single shift. Pat shocked him twenty of those times, not even thinking about it after the first dozen or so. He was a thirty-three-year-old electrician, which seemed appropriate. That was seventeen years ago. As of five years ago, she knew he was still alive.

By the time she moved on from that unit, Pat felt she could handle anything.

*

The hyperbaric oxygen chamber looks like a submarine inside, wide enough to contain two rows of gurneys against the walls with a narrow staff walkway between. Treatment gadgetry lines the walls—oxygen outlets, clasps for hanging IV bags. There are wall phones and an intercom system to communicate with the outside operator, who can also observe through portholes.

The idea is to simulate compression to higher atmospheric

pressures, such as are experienced with deep-sea diving, by delivering 100 percent oxygen. This leads to greater revascularization of injured bodily tissue. The chamber has two sides: a surgical side and a therapy side. Originally, it was devised with surgery in mind, but numerous other uses have been added with time and experimentation. Today, it is commonly used for patients with gas gangrene, an often deadly outcome of trauma, or large soft-tissue loss, such as degloving injuries experienced when someone is thrown from a motorcycle.

During "dives," a patient is brought down to a proper "depth," gauged on Navy diving tables, to facilitate therapy. The patient is wearing a clear plastic head mask that looks like something out of *Buck Rogers*. It is attached to an oxygen hookup that brings 100 percent oxygen. The nurse's job is to monitor vital signs and make sure everything is okay. It is she who is diving "normal," experiencing the pressure increase.

What Peggy likes about the chamber is sealing off the door and being alone with her patient. In the beginning, a doctor would go along on dives, but it became clear that there wasn't anything for him to do.

Routine dives for gangrene are 90 feet and take about ten minutes to compress. For air embolism, the depth would be 112 feet. If the patient was unconscious and awoke, they would stop there. If not, they would go to greater depth until the person woke up. She took one patient with hip pain down to 115 feet, where his pain disappeared (the nitrogen bubbles blocking blood flow having dissolved), then sat there as long as the diving tables instructed before decompressing.

Working alone can have its drawbacks. Peggy went to depth once with a woman who was a Jehovah's Witness and had refused blood transfusions for her massive GI bleed. She had a hemoglobin of three when the normal female range is twelve to sixteen. There's not much, other than a transfusion, that can help that, but she refused. It was postulated that if she was taken down, what oxygen she got could better circulate to cells.

She was put in inflated MAST trousers, designed to compress

the lower part of the body so that blood goes to the vital organs. It is necessary when compressing to watch air bags or the cup on an endotracheal tube, because the air drops and the cup needs to be re-inflated. That became a problem with the MAST trousers also. The air molecules compressed, and the trousers deflated.

Peg was pumping them back up when the woman went into cardiac arrest. She called for help to the outside operator, who immediately began to reverse compression, but it would take several minutes. Peggy had to try to handle several things simultaneously. It was like a sick joke, a crisis pantomime, administering amps of epinephrine and sodium bicarb, alternating with CPR and trying to re-inflate the trousers. It seemed as if she had one foot on the pump, one foot on the chest, and was injecting at the same time.

A new team of doctors and another nurse were brought into the other chamber and dove to meet her halfway so they could switch. Still, the woman died.

*

Mary Beth was taking care of a thirty-one-year-old with pancreatitis on SICU. He was one of the ugliest physical specimens she'd ever seen, with a face out of place anywhere but behind prison bars. He'd drunk and drugged himself into a state of bad, bad health. He had alcoholic hallucinosis and never even knew what day it was. His liver was garbage. He had abdominal ascites so pronounced that Mary Beth couldn't put a Texas catheter on his penis because she couldn't find it. But he was a sweetheart. They called him Bronco Billy because he'd whoop and roar, standing naked in the halls singing at the top of his lungs.

The surgical team would take him up to the OR, and all they'd do was put superficial incisions in his abdomen. This poor sucker had about eighteen draining superficial abdominal incisions, all draining pus. He had no family, never had a visitor. Whenever Mary Beth saw his doctor, she was sure to ask, "Are you sure you want us to code this man?"

She wanted to spit every time he said, "Yes."

He was resuscitated twice, paddled, and pounded on, acquiring rib-stress fractures for the two remaining days of his life. Mary Beth took him to the solarium for his last cigarette the day before he slipped into a coma and died.

*

"When you work with monitors, you think you have to have your eyeball on them constantly. You realize there should be somebody doing that, but there isn't. We've kind of grown comfortable on telemetry because we don't get into that many crises. If you're working with somebody who you think is in impending crisis, you're more attuned. Otherwise, it's a surprise to everyone if somebody goes bad. Of course, there's always that surprise."

*

It's not uncommon that during Cathy's twelve-hour day shift on the step-down unit, she will have a turnover of three or four of her five patients. It's a constant shuffle. She has to ship them to another floor or send them home, getting a replacement patient almost immediately. The average length of stay is twenty-four to seventy-two hours. Some will stay a week. Usually they are critically ill. They come from the coronary ICU, bypass patients, sometimes within twelve hours of surgery, with multiple lines, chest tubes, and pacemakers.

As each patient arrives, he is set up on a monitor to determine his base-line rhythm. Generally, once that is established, there isn't a lot to do for him unless an arrhythmia or chest pain develops. Then she has to pay attention. Mostly the patients on telemetry are walkie-talkies, up and able to care for themselves, unless problems start. When that occurs, she has to stop whatever else she is doing and deal with the problem, one on one, until it is resolved. Having one patient go bad means she has to ignore the other four—skipping regular meds and ACCU checks, food and dressing changes—which can be frustrating.

With thirty beds and six nurses, more than one patient may have difficulty at the same time, in which case she hopes the charge nurse is free and can help out. Otherwise, she skips room to room and hopes she can cover it all.

Usually she can get a chest pain resolved within thirty minutes, unless it develops into an MI. Then it can take an hour or two to get them stable and transferred to ICU. When someone does have an MI, everyone drops what they're doing and comes running to help. It's harder when the patient doesn't code but just gets very marginal. Then Cathy can't call the Code Blue Team. She is ever hopeful that there are enough nurses free to help out.

"What happens when there aren't enough?" she asked.

"Well, then," her nurse manager has told her, "you just better handle it alone."

It only happened once, when the patient/nurse ratio was too high. When she took the job, she was guaranteed a four to one ratio. It has inched upward on some shifts to six to one.

From what Cathy can judge, the turnover rate is far more important than the patients. If telemetry doesn't turn over, the ICUs back up, retarding the turnover from OR recovery or the ER. They can close the ER, but if someone out on a floor has a heart attack and needs an ICU bed, then ICU needs to push one of their patients onto telemetry, who has to push someone onto a floor or out the door. Everyone then hopes the patient sent out doesn't wind up back in the ER because they were sent out too soon.

*

The ICU is a symphony of stainless steel and machinery, holding hope and horror for all admitted. It is the symbol of science, the denial of decay. At its best, it is the finest medicine has to offer, swift intervention to save a life. At its worst, it is not so much life preserved as dying prolonged.

Sometimes Doris knows it's hopeless from the start: the eighty-five-year-old woman with a cancer-saturated system who fell down the stairs and has a subdural hematoma, blood seeping into the protective sac surrounding her brain. It's been four days, and she is still bleeding out from the subdural. Brain damage is assured if she lives. Still, the family wants her saved, the doctor wants to operate.

The lights are never turned off. In this windowless place where it's always "now," sensory- and stimuli-deprived patients have been known to lapse into confusion, "ICU psychosis," floating in a haze of medication, pain, and fear, necessitating being bound to their bed frame with soft cotton restraints.

The unit has eight, glass-enclosed rooms. Patient privacy and infection control are much better than older units, where beds were clustered in a circle about a nurses' station, separated only by curtains. Each room has a monitor overhead able to give EKG readings, Swan-Ganz line readings, arterial line, and intercranial pressure if needed.

Suction equipment and an oxygen adapter protrude from the wall beside a blood pressure device. Numerous drip lines hang at the head of each bed, rubbery IV bags with tubing descending through IVAC machines with digital readouts of drip factors, a peep alarm sounding should fluid backup occur. There may be a nitro drip for pain control, a dobutamine drip to help cardiac contractions, an antibiotic drip, a combo KVO (keep vein open) hydration/nutrition drip, and several other combinations, delivered straight or "piggybacked."

Much of the equipment is described by its manufacturers as "smart," able to adjust to the needs of users. Alarms exist on most equipment to alert the nurse to irregularities. Even the alarms on the equipment are smart. Smart and uniformly annoying: ventilators beep when interrupted for suctioning and honk for pulmonary pressure changes, such as when a patient coughs; monitors bong, and loudly when a deviation in systolic blood pressure occurs. That indicates a problem in cardiac pumping and grabs everyone's attention. The joke term for all this apparatus is "cardware."

Even the beds are smart today. There are a variety of multi-positional mattress types, air-cushioned to help prevent friction and skin breakdown, absorbent surface material, and removable wood-grain headboards that can be wedged beneath the back of a coding patient for CPR support. There are beds with automatic-digital patient weight readouts, and exit and weight shift alarms.

*

This whole week it's been just one thing after another. Someone has died every night of the week, people coding left and right. Doris hates it when someone's family is present when the patient codes, those mothers standing there while she pounds on their child's chest.

Horrendous, ungodly things have been happening. One patient was a lady who received the wrong blood. She bled all night long, oozed out, and proceeded to die. Nobody wanted to code her because nobody wanted his name on her chart. Everybody knew her case was going to court.

There was another guy who had to have a needle inserted in his head to relieve the pressure. He died, too. One patient was a twenty-one-year-old girl. A suicide. She had a big closet at home with a lot of shelves. She crawled up onto the top shelf and shot herself. The family had to tear it apart to get to her. One whole side of her face was caved in. Her skin grew gummy and gray. She took a long time to die.

Some patients take a long time to die.

There was an eighteen-year-old who came in for a hernia repair. The floor nurse told Doris he was a nice, bright kid. An athlete. He coded on the OR table. Transferred to ICU, he lived for six weeks on a vent, displaying all the signs of brain-stem dysfunction—absent pupillary light reflex, no gag reflex, no spontaneous respirations, "doll's eyes response." He was anoxic, not getting enough oxygen to his cells, because his brain was squashed and his body actually started deteriorating while being kept alive for so long on the machines. By the time he died, his skin was bluish and mottled. He looked like a skeleton lying in his bed.

Sometimes at night, Doris would walk past his room, and it would give her chills. With the dimmer lights on, it looked like he glowed.

There is a new grad being oriented to the unit who cries every night. Doris could set her watch by it; every night at 2:45 A.M. she calls her husband and by 3:00 she's in tears. Everybody is feeling the stress. Faces are stony. Nobody really looks at each other. Every day when she arrives for report, Doris asks, "Has it gotten any better?"

Every day she is told, "No."

*

The patient, Charlie C., had endstage multiple myeloma, cancer infiltration of bone marrow, and was in excruciating pain. His diagnosis had come late because he ignored earlier symptoms. Chemo and radiotherapy had had little effect. He was anemic, dehydrated, and in impending renal failure. By the time he became Diane's patient, he was obviously wasting, having lost several inches from his shrinking spinal cord.

When such patients start dying, they often have their pain worsened by severe spasms as muscle groups spontaneously grip tightly. It's extremely painful. His personal physician—possibly fearful of lawsuits, possibly attuned to some philosophical premise Di could never comprehend—didn't want to give Charlie any narcotics because it made him disoriented, even though he was endstage.

Charlie was on the unit for a week. He cried and begged for help almost ceaselessly. Initially, Di could get a resident to write for morphine, and Charlie would calm down for a time, only to resume as the pain reasserted itself. When the physician would arrive after Charlie had received some morphine and was disoriented, he'd say, "Nope, no more of that."

Soon the residents refused to cover because the attending was making angry noises about mismedicating his patient. The nursing supervisor took it up with the administrator, but nothing changed.

Di took to calling the physician at home in the middle of the night. When he refused to order narcotics, Di would be incensed.

"Listen to your patient," she would say, extending the receiver into the air. "The other patients in the unit are freaking out. The family was here this evening and were hysterical listening to him weep and plead, 'Help me! Help me!' "

The physician held his ground, ordering something like Darvocet, which everyone knew didn't do a damn bit of good. It got to the point where Diane didn't want to take care of the patient, frustrated with fighting and heartbroken with not being able to intervene, the powerlessness tasting like poison. But no one else could stand it either, so Charlie became hers again.

On the last day and a half of his life, Charlie started having seizures. Diane again called his doctor.

"You've got to order something. It's horrible here. The man is dying."

"It's not a nurse's job to make such pronouncements."

"He's groaning and screaming and seizing and twitching. He needs relief."

"All right, fine, give him five milligrams of Valium, IM."

"IM?" she nearly shrieked in disbelief. "IV would be quicker and more effective. He's already got the lines—why torture him with more needle sticks? What about a morphine drip?"

"Absolutely not. I'm not about to compromise his respiratory system. It's IM or nothing."

She administered the injections for the first few doses, each shot bringing moans and tears before a drowsy respite and whimpered thanks. But even before the specified minimum interval for doses had elapsed, the pain would eat through to his nerves again.

Diane hated the doctor and implied to the family that less than adequate treatment was just as negligent as outright mismanagement. She hated the hospital that supported the physician's turf in making all decisions. She hated feeling forced into making decisions that transgressed her ethical code. She decided on a highly illegal option—injecting the Valium directly into Charlie's IV port and charting it as given IM. It soothed his cries, allowing sleep. She followed this procedure for her two remaining shifts with Charlie, twenty-four of the final forty-eight hours of his life.

*

Peggy began pondering the implications of her work several months into her career. She was taking care of an older woman with gas gangrene and total body failure—renal failure, for which she was receiving dialysis, hepatic failure, pulmonary failure. She was on a ventilator, comatose. At the same time, Peggy was caring for a healthy young man who had been in a motorcycle accident. His brain was gone. They were in beds beside each other. There was very little chance of either ever regaining a meaningful life. Peggy graded their responses on the Glasgow Coma Scale. Why keep them going on respirators, costing thousands upon thousands of dollars, draining the family financially and emotionally? With each gurgle of the suction catheter, she wondered what the point was.

Her father's death helped her work the issue through. He was diagnosed with neck CA. The doctor wanted to do radical neck surgery, but her father refused. The surgeon was very straight-forward.

"He can have surgery and spend six months in an ICU with half a face and not be able to eat anything, or you can take him home and care for him there."

He died at home with the family.

It brought home the whole issue of quality of life.

*

Normally, on the cancer research ICU, what happens is this: somebody with leukemia arrives in septic shock, his pressure dropping. He ends up intubated, maybe on dialysis. But often they can be saved and go home and get through it. Most cancer centers focus on more general medical kinds of units, and the specialization isn't there. But if someone has cancer and needs an ICU, he needs to be with somebody who knows how to handle cancer. It's an intense environment. The families are all afraid that this person is going to die. The person is always afraid.

Marguerite often has patients look at her and ask, "Am I gonna die?"

"Well, no," she tells them. "Not today."

*

Confused patients are the ones Cathy finds most difficult. She hates to walk into a cubicle, find every tube yanked out, and the patient lying on the floor. She hates depersonalizing people by strapping them into a restraining vest, but that's the best she has to protect them. Some shifts it seems like there aren't enough Poseys in the world.

Some nurses are very solicitous with confused patients, but these people are disoriented and can't be communicated with. Cathy prefers to simply make certain the patient is safe, tie him in as tightly and securely as possible, and leave him alone.

Cathy has watched nurses try to talk patients into getting back into bed for an hour, telling them all the reasons they need to do so, which the patients forget before the sentence is complete. She has witnessed nurses agitate a patient with logic, turning a passive, directable, confused patient into an agitated, combative, confused patient.

All this with IV alarms going off, tube feedings to be done, and a tech on the phone bitching about a patient who hasn't gotten down to X ray. It can be an incredible pressure.

*

The man was found unconscious on the street, no social or medical history known. He was unresponsive to all but painful stimuli. He was a big guy, about six feet four, bald and muscular, diagnosed with sudden onset respiratory distress, though the ER doctor couldn't figure out why. After coding in the ER, Mr. A. was transferred to ICU.

Day shift had put soft cotton restraints on him. He had occasional bouts of thrashing confusion when he kept trying to tug out his endotracheal tube. He'd had some moments when he regained consciousness, but during the early evening shift, he slept soundly. When she returned from her dinner break, Maureen found he had pulled loose from the restraint and extubated himself. Mucus smeared both bed sheets and gown. Mucus glistened on the endotracheal tube beside him.

"Oh, Mr. A.," Maureen chattered. "Why did you go and do that? I told you it would just be for tonight. We'll have that tube out in the morning."

His best response was "Uggg," his eyes lolling, lips gapped.

As she cleaned him up, trying to avoid leaning into the mucus on the bed, she noticed that his fingernail glistened. Thinking he'd gotten mucus on his hand, she tried wiping it off when she realized it was nail polish. Looking closer, she noticed his well-manicured, high-gloss nails—not that it meant he was gay, but she felt the apprehensive AIDS-alert framework forming: "Well, just *may*be . . ."

He had a tattoo of an insignia on his arm that she turned to inspect when she spied the needle tracks. His sudden respiratory problems were becoming less of a mystery to Maureen.

She cleaned and re-situated him, doing a quick physical assessment, and reapplied the cotton restraints. He still had an IV line in his arm, which Maureen didn't want extracted, and a Dinamap blood pressure cuff on his arm. A Dinamap is a hefty boxlike machine that can be placed on a bedside table or its own portable stand. It has a timer that can be set to monitor blood pressure, heart rate, and mean arterial pressure on a schedule set anywhere from three- to ninety-minute intervals. A printout records each reading.

An hour or so later, Maureen was walking to another patient's room to answer a call light when she heard a crash from Mr. A.'s room. She scurried across the unit into his room. Sure enough, he'd gotten loose of the restraints and obviously decided to go to the bathroom, climbing over the bed rails and lugging the Dinamap behind him.

He'd apparently decided not to take the IV, though it was much lighter than the Dinamap and on a mobile pole. He'd bitten through the tubing, and it was a clean bite, too, not all stretched and tugged. Why he didn't just pull it out, she could only guess: the crazy dude—maybe when he awoke, he thought *that's* what was tying him to the bed. She wished he had just yanked it out because the jumbo 20-gauge needle still sticking out of his upper arm was shooting blood out wherever he moved. He had big veins, too, the kind Maureen prays for when she has to draw blood.

Dinamaps have a long cord and a long cuff. He'd dragged it the entire length of the double room. When a Dinamap malfunctions, it plays a mechanized tune, like an alarm. When Maureen entered the room, it looked like the bathroom scene from *Psycho*, blood splattered everywhere, light sprays where he'd moved quickly, puddles where he'd paused. At first she stood rooted, afraid to move, taking in the spectacle, the Dinamap tune repeating.

The needle was in his right arm, and he must have been righthanded because the bathroom door handle was dripping with blood. She was hesitant to open it. She patted her pockets for a pair of gloves and cursed herself when she found none. The door was ajar, the Dinamap's cord jamming it. Maureen touched a clean spot and inched it open.

He sat on the toilet, his jaw resting in his bloodied hand. Everything was bloody—the sink, the bathtub, the walls. It was dripping down into a puddle around the base of the toilet and the soles of his feet. She remembered the shiny nails and needle tracks, thinking, I don't get paid enough for this. She was thinking of it not as blood, but as AIDS—the bed is soaked in AIDS, there's AIDS all over the floor, AIDS dripping from the sink. I know what I should be doing, but I have to walk through AIDS to get to him.

"Oh, my God," a new nurse gasped behind her. "Let's get him out of there."

"Hold it." Maureen grabbed her elbow. "I'm not touching that sucker. Go get some gloves, several pairs. And a mask and goggles and some hemastats."

"Thank God, I'm a mature enough nurse to know that people rarely die from blood seeping from their IV site—because I wasn't touching it. Had this been five years ago, I'd have grabbed it and clamped it off with my hand, and have in fact done so. But no more. You're standing there remembering all the cuticles in your hand, the splinter you got the day before, how chapped your lips are. All that info just goes: *Wham, Wham, Wham!* in your head. You're thinking: This is AIDS! This is the real stuff.''

*

Peggy is much more aware of the patients she cared for six to a dozen years ago than the ones she cares for today. They now say the AIDS incubation period may last that long. She can remember many times having her hands in a patient's chest, doing manual heart massage with blood all over her. She recalls it being common to change scrubs two or three times a shift because they were saturated with blood. In the OR or trauma admitting that was the norm.

*

It's been over a year since Renee was stuck with a needle she had just removed from the arm of an AIDS patient. It was her first and only needle stick. The patient was a physician who had become infected when he was stuck by an AIDS needle. The patient did not know Renee had been stuck and was not told, there being no point in layering that guilt onto his suffering.

In the second the needle pierced her skin, every regret she'd ever hosted sprang to mind: I wish I'd . . . Why didn't I ever . . . She was working overtime, the end of her third twelve-hour shift that week, and was already tired. Now she was terrified.

First, she told her head nurse, who contacted the shift supervisor, who sent her to the ER for a tetanus shot. Renee protested this procedure—''It's not like I was bitten by a dog or stepped on a nail''—but didn't want to get into an argument, feeling she might easily lose control. She was extremely distressed but maintained her composure and completed her shift.

The next day, she had to come in early for an examination, to begin filling out the first of hundreds of forms and have the first blood drawn. For three months, blood was drawn every week. Thereafter, every month.

She became ill with a severe cough and fatigue. She was

started on AZT as part of a trial study examining the possibility of avoiding infection in those exposed through accidental needle sticks. The side effects started making her increasingly sick. She experienced caustic taste changes leading to anorexia. Food smells became particularly unbearable. Her hands would itch for hours, no matter how much lotion she applied. Insomnia was common—not only was it necessary to take the pills precisely every four hours, around the clock, interfering with the sleep cycle, but the drug kept her from dropping into the deeper stages of sleep, accentuating the mild confusional side effects as well. The fatigue was like a wall she could never get over. She found she needed to slow down all her actions, doubtful of her decisions. Something like figuring out the flow rate for a dopamine IV drip became an exercise in repetitive calculation.

Many things began falling apart in her life. She experienced little support at work. No allowances were made in her work load. She started being excluded by some co-workers, could feel people pull away as she entered an elevator. Some stopped talking to her. She sensed that others were more abrupt with her, angry that she'd somehow endangered them, or communicated a sense that she'd gotten herself into this fix because of her work habits—"That Renee, she's always getting so involved with her patients. . . . *Now* look what's happened to her."

Instances of outright hostility occurred. One nurse actually said, "I'm not gonna sit next to you anymore." A doctor whom she'd considered a friend became enraged when he saw her sitting in the clinic awaiting blood work one day.

"What are you doing here?" he hissed. "People can see you sitting here. What're you, trying to broadcast this?"

He has yet to speak to her since.

Her personal life suffered. A romantic relationship strained, snapped, and shattered. She became afraid to be around friends, afraid to have anybody touch her as if, against all rational awareness, she might give it to them. Some were supportive. Knowing her near-phobic regard for dirty hair and pallor, one nurse said,

"Well, Renee, if you do get sick, don't worry, I'll come and wash your hair and put your blush on."

All blood-work results thus far have been negative. Renee will be followed for possible infection for a year and a half. It is standard belief that if someone makes it to the three-month mark without seroconversion, they will be all right. Still, it's always in the back of her mind, What if I'm a late converter? What if they're wrong? What then?

*

It's the patients who fill Peggy back up, taking care of those who don't know how to take care of themselves. There are the little notes that a patient will scribble when he or she has an endotracheal tube in and can't talk.

Peg,
I don't want to get better because I'll lose you.

Love,

——

Children are hardest for her to deal with. She hates to see them hurt. She can justify a bit more pain in those her own age, having a car accident, injured in a fall. She hates to see kids broken into reality, to see frivolity and inquisitiveness squashed. She cared for a young girl once who hit a pothole on her bike and was thrown onto one of the handlebars, impaling it in her stomach. The girl never rode another bike.

A life is changed by bodily damage, perceptions, attitudes. Peggy has seen kids go back to high school or college altered in more than physique. Some make appointments to return to the clinic to speak with her.

"I don't fit in. Things just aren't the same, Peg."

"You're right, they're not the same. You're not the same. You've been through something none of your friends have. You know something they never will. Don't let it defeat you. You were strong enough to heal, you're strong enough to adapt."

Peggy uses the water to escape. Her house is within sight of the bay, surrounded by pine trees, a picnic bench in the side yard. She runs five miles along the shore each day. Then she goes to work for eight to twelve hours in a unit without windows. She is unsure she could do it without the water. She likes rowing and sculling and waterskiing. She has seven boats, none in perfect repair. She likes being kept busy working on them.

Friends tell her she should open a waterskiing school or charter the boats. She fears that combining the water with a job would remove its specialness. When she took her job at the university, staff members had the option of early retirement. She could have done so at age forty-three. When the university restructured a year ago, she lost that option. She's looking at several more years before she can work on her boats full-time.

"That doesn't appeal to me a bit. This place will be paid off in five years. I'm thinking about going part-time. I don't thrive in luxury and can probably get by without all the conveniences that full-time work would afford me. I'm thinking that after all these years of taking care of somebody else that if I don't start taking care of myself more, it'll all just be gone."

11

"No Lack of Choices"

Nursing Administration

Bill is the director of nursing (DON) of a university-based, regional child-development center. It is a relatively small facility in an active urban setting. The neighboring university boasts one of the oldest nursing schools in the country. The same is true for the medical school. In addition to its focus on service to handicapped children, the hospital also provides strong research, teaching, and training components. Bill is involved in all of these along with developing community programs with the state.

The patients' ages range from early childhood to adolescence. Developmentally, most are at the preschool level. Pediatric care has been the focus of Bill's career almost from the start. Most of it has been with children who have developmental problems. In nursing grad school, he happened to be in the right place when a traineeship in that speciality became available in Denver.

In an acute-care hospital, a child may come in with pneumonia, is treated, cured, and leaves. In this hospital, it is a much slower, less dramatic process. A child arrives with multiple handicaps that will never be cured. At best, he leaves with better motor skills so that he can clean and feed himself or walk better. He may also have improved his self-image and family relationships.

Bill doesn't consider himself to have a religion. He has a

strong leaning toward an existential view of life, trying to deal in a rational manner with the irrational circumstances of living. He found that if there is a single area where tragedies occur for no explainable, rational reason, it's when children are born with handicaps. Doing this work is an attempt to enter the realm of that absurdity and make the best of it. Robert Louis Stevenson once said, "Life's not a matter of holding good cards, but of playing a poor hand well." Bill thinks that is very relevant to his kind of work.

The kids who create the most anxiety in him are those he sees who are not born with handicaps, but who were normal, healthy kids until devastated by a tragic accident or illness. It hits too close to home. He has a daughter who is perfectly healthy, and such patients demonstrate how vulnerable we all are. Recently, a six-year-old girl was admitted. She had been in a car crash. There is little hope she'll escape being a quadriplegic for the remainder of her life—just because somebody made a wrong turn.

Most hospitals have numerous committee structures of which the director of nursing—more and more frequently termed vice president for patient care—is a member. The Committees are both within the nursing department and overlapping with others—administrative, medical, and nursing quality review committees; clinical risk management; patient classification; and medical staff committees; the forms, medical records and standards committees. The Joint Commission mandates that the DON be a member of many of these as well as other committees.

Because nursing departments are budgetary behemoths, climbing well into the millions of dollars, numerous layers of fiscal oversight are mandated, the buck stopping at the DON's desk. At least one day each week is spent on budgetary concerns alone. In a survey done by the American Organization of Nurse Executives and published in the December 1989 *American Journal of Nursing*, the profile of a senior nurse executive in a hospital with 250 beds or more was typified as being a forty-five-year-old female who is married with two children. Holding a master's degree, she likely works fifty-five-hour weeks and manages a nursing budget of $29 million, or 30 percent of the total hospital budget. Salaries for such positions have been reported to run as high as $170,000, but according to a 1990 American Hospital Association survey, the typical range for a nursing vice president is from $45,000 to $86,000.

As with almost all directors of nursing, Bill is not involved directly in the clinical realm. But for the last two years, he has chaired the hospital's Human Rights Committee, which exists to render technical assistance, through policy and procedural formation, to all staff members about ethical issues. Recently AIDS has been a focus of much discussion—dealing not only with infection-control issues, but issues of confidentiality, staff anxiety, and testing. Thus far no blanket testing has occurred, though tests are done on a case-by-case basis, if there is any indication the child might be positive.

Recurring ethical issues usually revolve around the topics of behavior management and the use of restraints on otherwise uncontrollable patients. The hospital employs a strong behavior-management program based upon behavioral principles, rewarding positive behaviors and discouraging negative ones. For some children, that has meant the use of types of aversive stimuli, such as a water gun. Developmentally impaired children sometimes exhibit serious self-injurious behaviors, head banging or punching themselves in the face, biting a hand until it is welted and raw. When all else fails, a mildly adverse action, such as a water squirt in the face, administered when the behavior is occurring, has been shown to make a difference.

The hospital employs fifteen separate disciplines; name it and it's there: medicine, nursing, social work, movement therapy, speech therapy, psychology, pharmacy, nutrition, etc. By its nature, the entire system is interdisciplinary. Bill sees functioning in a truly interdisciplinary manner as a goal to be approached rather than achieved. Certain situations are very open and collaborative. Others are very territorial.

The greatest challenge he perceives for nursing has to do with the profession's image, how outsiders view nurses. Nurses are unable to float along on their credentials. New physicians can come, and simply by virtue of that title, a certain amount of positive expectation and regard exists for them. This is true with other therapists as well.

Nurses, however, are constantly having to prove themselves. If there is something innovative and exciting that nursing wants to implement, it must be demonstrated thoroughly before being accepted. People just assume that nurses don't do those kinds of things.

Conflicts are common with new employees who arrive with the idea that nurses exist only to carry out their directives. At Bill's hospital, when a child is cared for, even routine ADLs (activities of daily living: hygiene, toileting, etc.), and certain protocols must be maintained. For instance, when a child with oral-motor deficits is fed or being put to bed, the child must be handled in accordance with physical therapy protocols. When dealing with behavioral-management issues, there are psychological protocols.

Experienced nurses practicing in a professional manner don't just passively accept protocols from other disciplines. Those nurses make it clear they are not here simply to change diapers and get the kid looking shipshape. Bill considers himself a proactive nursing administrator and encourages his staff to interact with specialists to arrive at the protocol that is best suited for the specific needs of that child as well as that therapy.

There was an instance where a physical therapist decided to position a child in a certain way, but that position compromised the child's circulatory status. His nurse had to intervene and work out a protocol that addressed more than a single aspect of treatment. It is all too easy for treatment to get focused on the needs of a discipline rather than the needs of the patient. Bill believes that is where nursing, with its holistic overview, has the strongest role to play.

Though his master's degree is in nursing, Bill does not feel focused entirely in that area. His interest in developmental disabilities transcends nursing's impact on treatment, extending into the realm of entire programs. His doctorate will be in Public Health Administration. It is an interdisciplinary degree program with other nurses, physicians, social workers, and even lawyers and MBAs enrolled.

Bill is very protective of his nursing identity, though, believing it allows him a more global perspective than most other professionals have when examining programs. Essentially, it goes back to the nursing perspective—not looking at a particular body system or a single need, but seeing a whole person. That translates nicely when it comes to setting up a multifaceted program and understanding how it impacts on whole people, not only someone's cystic fibrosis or birth defect.

Bill's first position as a new nurse was about as far from dealing with innocent children as can be imagined. He was one-third of a practice—along with a physician and a family nurse practitioner—contracted to develop a health care system for a county prison. He was involved in the program's planning and development, as well as working in a hands-on capacity. It was three months of hell, a true nightmare experience.

There were constant drug seeking and other manipulative behaviors on the part of the inmates. The experience pointed out to him just how vulnerable he could be while having no awareness of danger. He would be in the midst of situations like being in a prisoner's cell without the benefit of backup, arguing with him, informing him sternly, "No, you can't get this medication because it's not ordered for you."

Initially he possessed a sense—never clearly articulated to himself—that because he was there in the name of good, he was in some vague way protected. . . .

"Nobody'll harm me. I'm here to help."

He was right out of nursing school and very much into dealing with "whole people" and "the power of touch"—the whole holistic nursing school agenda. He recalls sitting with prisoners in the infirmary, touching their hands, their knees, whatever it

took to convey a sense of trust, openness. Later, he would ruminate: "Good God, what message must you have been sending?" When things started getting weird with the guards (many
of them were later indicted for drug dealing and other infrac-
tions), he'd sit back at night and realize just *how* vulnerable he'd
been. Then it started getting scary. He started doubting his judgment, developing an almost paranoid feeling that he couldn't
trust the world.

One man was imprisoned because he'd murdered his young
son. Here was Bill trying to engage him in a relationship, to
forge a therapeutic alliance. The man would hardly ever talk to
anyone, but he had a poster on his bedside. It was a side view
of a big, open field with what looked like a tusk sticking up out
of the ground. Observed from just the surface in the picture, the
aboveground, it was impossible to tell what it was. But seen in
its entirety, the picture revealed that the tusk was attached to a
gigantic, ugly monster crouching underground.

The picture showed a tractor coming to remove it.

The caption read: "Sometimes it's best to leave well enough
alone."

It was always like swimming upstream, trying to get something positive going; but the odds against them were staggering.
The final straw was a break-in at the infirmary. A lot of drugs
were stolen, and there was a couple of overdoses. A guard had
given an inmate the key. Bill and his associates recognized the
need to relinquish the contract.

Staffing the nursing department of Bill's present facility has been
a constant, day-to-day struggle. Because his is a small, very
specialized facility, Bill feels the impact of the nursing shortage
acutely. He can recall a few years back when any advertised
vacancy brought in twenty responses. Recently, he has had to
rely on agency nurses a great deal and fears that quality of care
has been compromised in consequence. Agency nurses usually
only come for a few days at a stretch. It's a relief to find one
who will keep returning, even if only because they know where

things are located, though they often supply only the minimal energy necessary to get through a shift.

There have been some serious problems with agency nurses. One was supposed to administer 0.6 mg of atropine prior to a test. Instead she gave 6.0 mg. One would think she would have known something was amiss when she had to open ten vials; it comes packaged in unit doses for convenience, but that unit dose is the usual dose. She had to give three injections. Every nurse has made a med error, but that speaks to a new level of incompetence. The patient wound up in ICU with cardiac complications.

Still, the units have to be staffed. The Joint Commission recently cut its approval of Charity Hospital in New Orleans due to short staffing. Medicare allows a med error rate of no greater than 5 percent. And staffing shortages have been implicated in a number of lawsuits won against hospitals.

Bill sees the whole area of health care becoming increasingly contract-oriented. The solution to the shortage for many hospitals has been to enter bidding wars, offering bundles of money by converting benefits into cash the way agencies do. He scans the multiple nursing want-ad pages daily, keeping an eye on what others are offering. It's been hard to compete.

He finds a very different kind of nurse emerging—one who comes for the money. It's clear that individuals have differing levels of commitment to careers. For some, it is probably just an income. But that's true in any line of work; he knows doctors and lawyers who view patients and clients as a means to getting a new car or sending their kids through college. It's not that he thinks nurses don't deserve ample compensation for their work, but it is difficult to see his profession reflecting the consumer values of the larger society, the callous calculation mindful only of "What's in it for me?"

He has mixed feelings about the whole issue of appropriate compensation for nurses. On the one hand, someone can go to an associate-degree school for two years and be able to enter the market earning in the mid-to-upper $20,000 range. He sees that as not only reasonable, but a desirable opportunity for many young people. He knows individuals in other disciplines, like social work, with master's degrees who are making less.

On another level, he can look at the value of what nurses do, the responsibility nurses shoulder—the fact that a nurse may be responsible for the total well-being, even survival, of from one to over ten patients' lives on a daily basis, making critical decisions about what needs to be done to sustain those lives, knowing when to intervene and how—then the pay doesn't seem very reasonable. Particularly when he thinks that someone working in a grocery market may be making the same amount.

"There are those who say that in terms of the significance of what nurses do, we are just as important as physicians and should be paid at that level. I'm somewhat critical of that view. Our educational background is quite different. We don't make that commitment up front of eight to twelve or more years of our lives.

"Then, too, there's the issue of mobility within the profession. A lot of staff nurses complain there is nowhere to go, that there is little room for advancement. Other professions make most of their educational investment prior to practice, such as spending seven years becoming a lawyer before going to work. Nurses can enter the workplace earlier. But if they stay at the staff nurse level, career mobility can get limited in terms of salary increases.

"Variation can come in having the freedom to travel anywhere and get a job or switch around within areas of practice. There is certainly no lack of choices in nursing. But economically and powerwise, you stay within a narrow range.

"If you are willing to go back for further education, though, there are all kinds of other nursing levels—clinical specialist, nurse practitioner, midwives, nurse anesthetists, and administrative positions are all available. I see quite a breadth and depth of experience available. Financially, of course, you're not going to be in the same ballpark as engineers or lawyers—

people with basically the same educational commitment—but you certainly can make a living and have more control over your career.''

12

"Right up against Life"

Nurse-Midwives

Outside the United States, midwifery has been popular for centuries. In England, nurse-midwives deliver 70 percent of all babies born. In Norway, the figure is as high as 90 percent. Vera, who today practices in the Baltimore area, trained as a midwife in South Africa, where midwifery was common. Her career took her from there to England and America. Originally, her education consisted of a diploma with a midwifery certificate. Coming to America in 1967—and being foreign-trained, but not British-trained—she was unable to obtain certification for two years. Eventually she broke ground by becoming the first non-British-trained midwife accepted in the States.

She was drawn to midwifery because midwives are able to diagnose and treat, to counsel and teach. She despised the powerlessness of floor nursing, the lack of decision making. She wanted the independence of private practice.

Clients mainly come to her through word of mouth. Many are professionals: several nurse practitioners, teachers, a lot of lawyers, businesspeople. Many are having their second child and don't want any part of what happened to them in their first pregnancy—labor induced for dubious reasons, having little input into their care, often feeling trivialized and humiliated. They want to have more control over what's happening. Vera and her partners encourage that. Nonintervention unless needed is their philosophy.

Midwives care for healthy women from menarche through menopause, seeing them through all their active phases: the onset of sexual activity, marriage, children, contraception. It's a tremendous growth period. Vera enjoys the teaching part most of all, watching a person grow and learn. Helping someone change bad habits—such as talking a young, sexually active woman into modifying potentially harmful behavior, helping her find alternative ways to get the same needs met, and planning for her future—is a rich experience. It is a relationship that can be immeasurably satisfying. As is assisting someone with the passage into menopause. There is teaching at all levels and transitions, help to be offered today to make future periods easier and more productive.

Midwives don't treat abnormalities. Vera's midwifery group has an agreement with an obstetrician who sees their patients if a problem develops. If Vera finds an uncommonly large fibroid uterus, she will refer the woman. She had two patients with such large fibroids that it was impossible for them to deliver naturally. If a patient has an infection or STD (sexually transmitted disease), Vera will treat her unless she develops an abscess. If so, Vera refers.

Midwives don't do cesarean sections. Vera's patients who need to have a C-section book the procedure with the group's physician and then don't see him again. He is more of a consultant brought in to perform a specific task amid the support, encouragement, and instruction rendered by the midwife. Usually a patient needs a section if she has a small pelvis, proven with her first baby. Or if she had a previous emergency section and the cut was done wrong, she will require another. Vera accompanies her patient throughout the procedure, remaining with them through the recovery phase.

As recently as 1960, there were only three legal jurisdictions where certified nurse-midwives could practice. Today, CNMs practice in all fifty states in a variety of health care settings: hospitals, HMOs, public health departments, private practices. Roughly 85 percent of all deliveries attended to by a CNM are in hospitals, 11 percent in birthing centers, and the final 4 percent in homes. In 1987, according to the National Center for Health Studies, midwifery accounted for 98,425 babies (up from 19,425 in 1975) or 2.6 percent of all births nationwide. Twelve states reported 5 percent or more.

The clinical rotation Kay most hated in nursing school was obstetrics. But after graduation, she worked in one hospital for several years, trying out several departments, including OB, and to her surprise she found she liked it. Still, she never considered it a focus of potential practice.

She was married at that time, and her husband's grad-school placement required a relocation to South Carolina. There she decided to work in public health. The clinic she worked at performed all prenatal assessments, healthy maternal/child and OB care. The doctor saw each patient once. The clinic nurses followed them the rest of the time with a high degree of autonomy.

Kay was placed in charge of the "granny midwives" for the county. Most granny midwives were older women with no formal training. In South Carolina at that time, it was a traditional position, handed down from mother to daughter to granddaughter. But, in order to be registered with the state, each needed to attend classes to broaden her knowledge base and for evaluation of updated skills.

Kay stayed for four years, solidifying her area of expertise, her interest in women's health issues ever deepening. When she decided to pursue a master's degree, the choices fell between Maternal/Child Health and Nurse-Midwifery. Kay and her husband chose Emory University in Atlanta. It offered an excellent educational program for her and employment opportunity for him.

The midwifery program lasted a calendar year and a half, straight through the summer. It consisted of core courses in master's level work, theory, and research, progressing into women's health. There were lengthy clinical rotations, also. Far longer than for other tracks. Midwifery students were somewhat isolated from the rest of the students because there was so much clinical work. It was impossible for Kay to hold even a part-time job.

After all core courses were passed and all rotations finished, there was an ''integration period.'' Integration is a sort of mini-internship for midwives usually lasting about six to eight weeks. For her integration, Kay functioned as a staff nurse midwife, but with greater supervision. Because of her public health work, the transition to expanded responsibility presented no shocks. The only problem Kay had with the program was that she was also doing her thesis. It was a difficult period, juggling work, research, and writing, but Kay was very focused and thought it an excellent experience.

Katherine entered nursing specifically to become a midwife. At the age of thirteen, she met a nurse-midwife from England, a friend of her church pastor's wife, who told her enough about the profession to know that was what she wanted to do. Katherine initially graduated from an associate's-degree program and completed an RN-to-BSN degree while working in labor and delivery. At twenty-one, she entered the air force because it offered a midwifery program and helped with educational costs.

She qualified for a two-year master's midwifery program at the University of Utah, which provided a broad transcultural philosophical basis. There she spent a lot of her time working in the Native American culture, performing her integration in a birthing center on the Navajo reservation. The experience furnished her with a great deal of information about non-Euro approaches to birth—nutritional influences, positional variations, exercise, and pain suppression.

''The experience of Navajo women in labor is unique in how they express themselves. During the second stage of labor, when it's very painful, most women flail about and cry. I found with my Navajo patients that if I didn't tune in to tiny indications of second-stage discomfort—curling of toes or beads of sweat on the upper lip or brow—that I could easily miss the baby.''

The nurse-midwife Katherine was assigned to work with had delivered over five thousand babies on the reservation. Physician backup was mostly by general medical officers who tended to know less than the midwives. Consequently, there was a corresponding broadening of responsibility in dealing with fetal abnormalities. Postpartum hemorrhage was commonplace, producing more complications. Because alcoholism and diabetes are rampant among Indians and their glucose metabolism is extra sensitive, corresponding problems were also present. There were also instances of traditional healing, such as medicine men coming to perform rituals alongside those using Western methods. All of which Katherine learned to incorporate in solidifying her practice.

Approximately 4,000 certified nurse-midwives are currently licensed to practice in the United States. Since the early 1970s, 200 to 250 have been certified yearly. In 1987, according to a survey by the American College of Nurse-Midwives (ACNM), the mean annual ACNM income was $33,659. Most midwifery services are covered by private insurance carriers as well as Medicaid, Medicare, and CHAMPUS. The ACNM has a membership of roughly 2,900, boasting the highest percentage of Ph.D.s of any nursing speciality. Nationwide, there are twenty-seven accredited nurse-midwifery educational programs.

In 1979, when Kay moved to New Mexico and came to her current hospital, there were four nurse-midwives. Her caseload was divided between inpatient maternity work and an infant care project on a nearby air force base. In her ten-year tenure, the midwifery staff has expanded to ten, their practice sphere including the Indian Health Service. Kay is also a member of a private midwifery practice.

Midwives in the hospital clinic function within treatment protocols, a step-by-step formula dividing the progress of labor into antepartum, partum, and postpartum. Each phase has boundaries for independent midwife coverage, comanagement with a physician, or turning patients over to a physician. As long as treatment needs remain within the protocol, midwives do not have to consult a physician. When a consultation is required, midwives do so with third and fourth-year residents.

In Kay's facility, midwives fall under the School of Medicine. The faculty and department chair are very supportive of midwives, feeling it would be difficult to manage without them. OB residents come and go with the academic cycle. On the rare occasion when disagreements with residents arise that cannot be talked out between them, the department is very supportive. They recognize that the CNMs are the permanent people.

Normally, though, most problems can be sorted out. Kay is a great believer in keeping lines of communication open. In the clinical realm, she attempts to keep her backup physician apprised of all changes in her patient's condition, actual or potential (for instance, a patient at risk for a postpartum hemorrhage from a slack uterus caused by prolonged labor, a potentially profound problem). Kay will usually alert the physician about any concerns, even though it hasn't progressed to a comanagement phase.

"Just be forewarned. If I call for you, this may be what the problem is."

After graduation from her midwifery program, Katherine had four years of service to repay to the air force. Initially, she practiced in a military hospital, basically functioning as a resident. Anybody who arrived at the door was hers to care for during that shift. Later, she became involved in teaching and research, working on low technology methods that can be used by women in this country who don't have immediate access to electronic fetal-monitoring machines, or women in developing countries where there is poor electronic equipment. The goal is to identify babies who are at risk for antepartum death.

By the time Katherine had completed her payback period, a physician researcher colleague, a perinatologist, was offered a departmental chairmanship in a prestigious East Coast university hospital. As part of a package deal he structured with the institution, Katherine accompanied him. This hospital had phased out its midwifery program in 1981, and there was no joy expressed at having a CNM return to practice there, so Katherine planned to keep a low profile. The labor and delivery nurses were ecstatic to have a midwife on staff, but most of the physicians she encountered were very cool.

Soon after establishing herself, she received a call from a friend at the School of Hygiene who wanted to recommend a patient who had recently resettled from Mali, a republic in western Africa, with her husband, who was on a university fellowship.

"This woman's here and needs a birth attendant. I know that you can do real well with her, even though she doesn't speak English."

Two weeks later, this woman came in. She'd had ruptured membranes for a long time, and Katherine had to induce labor. The university has a large foreign-studies department, and Katherine was able to contact an ex-Peace Corps volunteer who spoke the French dialect of Mali to aid in communication.

Now, in Mali, women don't hang around in bed. After several fruitless attempts to cajole the woman into remaining in bed, Katherine relented and had the bed removed from the room. Having been trained in the birthing center, she found no position or request out of line. Unusual, maybe—like if someone wanted to take the placenta home to make a milk shake, but then the Navajo would take placentas home to bury all the time. Observers might think it strange, but . . .

Labor wound up being done with the woman on the floor with

a hands and knees delivery. From Katherine's standpoint, it was a beautiful birth.

"It's important to respect the woman's wishes and enhance her privacy, to accept whatever behavior she needs to express, to witness and foster that. If she wants to yell out, to accept that. You give permission for her to make it her experience in whatever form it takes.

"You can tell just at the moment that the baby is born that the woman's self-esteem about her role as a woman has been enhanced, despite the common humiliations in the process. To witness what can happen to women in the birth experience can be very moving."

Not everyone was as elated about the event, however. Individual reactions ran from aghast to disgusted. Someone was thoughtful enough to take pictures as evidence, lest the proper authorities doubt the descriptions. As word spread, the dominant opinion was: *This* is why we didn't want midwives and their bizarre methods in our institution.

One of the attendings cornered Katherine's boss, demanding an explanation.

"Have you heard what that midwife of yours did?"

"I know." He beamed. "Isn't it great? It's nice to see we're individualizing care to meet the needs of patients."

By the end of the week, the incident was written up in the hospital's staff paper, the article's focus being that individualized care had come to the halls of the hospital. Oh, blessed event.

Currently there is a trend in maternal/fetal medicine that Kay finds disturbing. The emerging idea is that everything is abnormal until proven otherwise. She sees a sharp increase in the use of invasive technology. Midwives stress that pregnancy is not an illness. Kay sees devices such as intrauterine pressure monitors to measure the strength of contractions internally being commonly abused. The results are accurate, but there are many disadvantages, including a high-infection risk.

Such things are used too often. People are rushed too much. There is little patience. If somebody comes in with ruptured membranes, but labor hasn't commenced, residents will give Pitocin to induce labor after a maximum of only six hours.

One of the things Kay most dislikes about monitors is that the patient is completely immobilized. Forced inactivity adds to the woman's sense of helplessness. It is diametrically opposed to the philosophy of nurse-midwifery. Labor doesn't progress as smoothly when the woman is immobilized. When she can move around, it progresses faster and the baby descends sooner. There is less discomfort, requiring less pain relief. There is less likelihood of needing a C-section or forceps delivery.

But if the patient is active, it is harder to monitor her. If there is a high-risk intervention in progress, such as giving Pit to induce labor, she can't possibly be off the monitor because fetal stress has been initiated. Then it is necessary to know how the child is every single minute.

The composition of Kay's private-practice clientele is telling. Two-thirds are medical personnel, mostly nurses, physicians, and their spouses. The nurses tend to be those from the more high-tech intensive care areas, those geared toward the most invasive patient management techniques. The physician group includes several obstetricians, the very people instructing residents in high-intensity interventionist OB techniques. For themselves, they prefer individualized care, choices, and control. They would rather not have a physician whose focus is on illness, viewing their own pregnancy as healthy and trusting Kay to refer if something is abnormal. Each group is open to the possibility of technological intervention, but not routinely.

The examination room is usually the first stop for an admission. It is the size of a large bathroom, and just as impersonal. An exam table with stirrups is crowded amid cabinets and supplies. Only the tiniest surface exists for charting.

It's common that a clinic patient will arrive at some off-hour believing she is in labor. Many times it's a false alarm, particularly for a first birth. Often she is sent home. If the woman is three or four centimeters dilated, or if her amniotic sac has ruptured, she will be told to stay. If a nurse-midwife is on duty, she'll be able to leave her gown on and walk around for a couple hours. Sometimes she protests this, being exhausted at that point from hours of contractions, but it's the healthiest thing for her. If one of the residents has received her, she'll probably be placed in bed and strapped to a monitor. Once that happens, the chances of getting back up are pretty slim.

Sometimes Katherine fills in for residents when they are short-staffed, pulling a twenty-four-hour shift on labor and delivery, either doing deliveries or just helping out in general. She has to keep in mind that she is there to serve as a stopgap and not introduce too heavy a midwifery philosophical emphasis. Also, the population being served from the surrounding neighborhood is very different from her private-practice patients, whom she has known for nine months—or three years and two deliveries—and whose course of labor she can better predict.

The walk-in group are likely to have had little or no prenatal care. There is a lot of drug abuse, women doing cocaine in the bathroom to get them through labor. Violent labors with placental eruptions from crack use are an everyday occurrence. There are many dead and damaged babies. Katherine sees a lot of judgmental interventions on the part of staff members: "Do you know what you've done to your baby?" She feels such comments have no meaning. It's like telling a teenage mother in labor pains, "Well, I guess you should remember this the next time you want to have sex."

She can understand the frustrations of staff members, residents, and nurses—she has delivered a mother who was thirteen years old—but she can't condone it. When hearing such remarks, she will take the person aside and express her displeasure with them.

"I try to treat each woman with respect, even if she is quite high or has done something dangerous to herself. You have to help them capture that moment. You can only hope that if you can convey that she has value, some of that may influence her future choices about how she'll treat herself and her child."

The hospital has several comfortable birthing rooms. The delivery is usually done in the room. A plush-cushioned couch occupies one wall. Family members are welcome to attend the birth experience. Along one counter are a hot plate for making tea or cocoa, a cooler for beverages. Room lights operate on a dimmer switch. Radio and TV are available. Emergency equipment is readily available, discreetly stored behind closet doors, except for the fetal-heart monitor, which is the size of a large TV and too cumbersome to conceal.

Colors in the birthing room are muted—light pastels, off-white, gray. There is a sense of coolness. The walls used to be covered in print wallpaper. It seemed cheerful at first, but after long hours of staring at the tiny print patterns, patients would complain it made them feel "zooy." And it was very hard to keep clean. Iodine and blood-splash stains wouldn't wash out.

The birthing bed affords several positional choices. A woman can lie or sit. There are supports for squatting. It can be converted quickly into a delivery bed if need be and theoretically turned into an OR table, though it's never been done, because of the objections of the anesthesia people.

There is the faintest odor of bleach in the air. It is comforting, reassuring, touching off associations with cleanliness. It is used as a virucide. "Universal precautions" have been instituted by most hospitals. Gloves, masks, gowns, and goggles are to be used whenever in a situation where one may come into contact with bodily fluids. And a birth scene can get very messy, with lots of blood and body fluids flying. Getting splashed in the face is not uncommon.

Plastic glasses are kept at the doorway of each room. They

are not as comfortable as goggles but are more readily accessible. If an emergency occurs and people get busy fast, someone takes responsibility for running around putting a pair on anyone who isn't wearing them. It makes for less intimacy with the patient, but no one complains anymore. Demographic studies indicate that the number of women with AIDS-infected babies is increasing sharply. This is a wave that is not expected to crest until the mid-nineties.

Kay sees her role as doing whatever is needed to safeguard mother and child. When hiring new CNMs, she is very specific that sitting with the patient throughout the delivery is part of the job. She knows midwives who enjoy the prenatal teaching phase, striking a bond with a new client, and doing deliveries, being the first to clasp each slithering new life, but who shy away from sitting with their patient from contraction to completion.

Patients were very appreciative of Kay because of her presence throughout, whether actively engaged with delivery techniques or sitting quitely in the corner, reading or doing needlework, during the lull times of labor.

Nurses often think they always have to be busy. One of the things Kay learned in her midwifery program was that it was all right just to sit in a room and be with the patient. There are times this becomes an issue with staff nurses. They see her sitting in the room having a cup of tea with the patient while it's crashingly crazy out on the floor, and they're wondering why she doesn't come and pitch in.

It's an individual perception. Other nurses will come into the room and sit for a minute amid the madness and join them, trying to soak in some of the peacefulness before returning to the floor.

Sometimes midwives have conflicts with staff RNs who are used to having more control, particularly in university settings where they are accustomed to instructing residents and interns in the early part of their practice. Kay, as nurse-midwifery service director, meets quarterly with unit charge nurses to smooth over misunderstandings or conflicts. With frequent staff turnover, there are recurring themes: one nurse complains she has to do the scut work for the CNMs; since they're nurses, she feels they should pull their own weight. Another staff nurse might be uncomfortable with Kay's method of not continuously monitoring fetal-heart tones or not routinely starting an IV. Another nurse may be apprehensive about a patient making a lot of noise, believing the woman should be snowed with pain meds.

But Kay encourages her patients to make as much noise as they wish rather than taking meds, not really caring if this woman straining to bring new life into the world is seen as "a good patient." She keeps a sign over her desk: "DON'T FLOAT THROUGH LIFE, MAKE WAVES."

It gets tiresome having to explain to new people coming on staff—be they nurses, faculty physicians, administrators, residents, hospital PR people—just what a nurse-midwife *is*. Having to justify that the practice is safe. Physicians don't have to do that. Each time someone arrives from a hospital where women are kept bed-bound, fully monitored, they assume that's the only safe way to have a baby. Then Kay has to go through the whole thing over again. All midwives deal with it, but because Kay is in an administrative position, it falls to her even more.

> "Some nurses—and sometimes I wish there were more—are able to have a holistic perspective and look at the psychological and emotional as well as the medical and managerial aspects of the work. Too often, though, that's forgotten in practice. And it's one of the most positive things a nurse brings to the work. We have become so busy trying to prove our worth in task competency that some of the art that brings humanity into focus is being lost."

Katherine's longest span attending a labor was thirty-nine hours. Usually shifts will change every twenty-four hours. Katherine will shorten the shift if she feels herself getting so burnt out that she can't make a good decision. Then she'll call in one of her partners to spell her while she catches some sleep.

"It's important to take each minute as it comes, staying tuned to the patient, observing and monitoring the environment and the progress. You might think it would be a big yawn, but it's very intense. It's a constant mental effort to go through the assessment of labor. It's exhausting, but there is a second-wind effect that takes place. I think I must go into a trance or something. It's as difficult to explain as it is for women who have been in labor that long to say how it is for them. It's almost a timelessness."

There are often others in the room that she needs to keep an eye on as well. There have been as many as twelve or fifteen people in a birthing room, which can get somewhat chaotic. But as long as everyone knows there is only one boss, it's okay.

Not long ago, she had a nurse who was in labor. This woman had expressed concern in earlier meetings about her mother's attendance at the birth. Her mother was quite religious, a charismatic Pentecostalist, but the daughter did not hold the same religious values. She was in nice active labor when the mother arrived. Soon the daughter was on her hands and knees praying with her.

Labor stopped.

Katherine had to ask the mother to step outside. First she conferred with her patient, by now in a frothy state of anxiety, and helped her calm down, sitting on the edge of the bed, rocking with her, soothingly stroking her back and shoulders, taking command. Next she spoke with the mother, inviting her back in with the stipulation that there were rules that needed to be adhered to. To which she agreed. Soon the labor resumed, and the baby was born without any complications.

Nurse-midwives oversee the care of their patients from the time they arrive. The focal word Kay likes to use is "choice." She strives to supply patients with many options, providing a sense of empowerment. Even if the choice is between lying on the right side or on the left, sitting here or there, it does allow for choice, rather than Kay saying, "Look here, you have to do this, and you have to do that."

Much of the time is spent on teaching and answering questions, reviewing the probable stages to come, encouraging the participation of the birth partner if one is present. Women entering labor share the same fears as any patient: Will I lose control? Will I be able to hold up?

Kay informs the mother what is happening at each step. Even if emergencies arise, she delegates what tasks she can to the staff nurses—call the physician, call anesthesia—so she can remain with her patient. Patients become overwhelmed simply because there is no one explaining things to them. People perform much better if there is some calm voice amid the swirl. Even if Kay is the only one available to perform emergency measures, she tries to keep the patients apprised and engaged, to be of support and reassurance to her, as well as role model for residents and nurses.

Giving birth is different from most hospital procedures. The patient not only has to cooperate but be actively engaged in order to have control and have it go well. She has a lot to do. When a woman is in transition, the second stage of labor, when she starts pushing, one of the things she often says is, "I can't do this anymore. I want somebody else to do this."

It's interesting to watch someone work that out. It can feel powerful to help someone go from feeling like that to realizing that there is no way out of this, that the way out is to go through it. And that she can go through it with some dignity and power, and be in touch with what's going on.

> "When a woman is thrashing around, yelling and screaming and having a hard time cooperating, she is not only experiencing pain and fear, but there is also something spiritual occurring. It has to do with being right up against life and death at the same time.

"It's not something that you can talk about in that setting, but being aware of it makes it possible to address the fear. It is a profound experience and can shift in a second from being the most wonderful moment to the most terrifying experience that a woman has ever had. Knowing that gives you a lot more patience."

When it goes well, when a woman can have this resource in herself, or be helped to find it, then having a baby can be one of the times when she feels the most powerful, particularly the prepared, healthy woman who has looked forward to this as a peak experience all her life. She can become the most in touch with what she can do, both with her body and with her will.

Of course, sometimes things can go wrong without forewarning. One of Katherine's first deliveries at the military hospital was that of a Japanese woman whose husband was in the air force. Katherine had just come on shift and met the patient when the baby was due. She delivered an at-term child with very severe abnormalities—lower limb deformities, holes in the diaphragm—who died twenty minutes later.

Observing the mother was a striking experience for Katherine. Because of her Japanese cultural norms, her reaction was different from what was expected. She was more subdued, but not blocked from her grief. Having had the Navajo experience, Katherine could recognize the difference while the husband, a midwestern American, was having his more overt response to the torment of loss. It was very moving, being a party to that, retrieving the baby from the OR, where it had been whisked off to in an attempt to forestall his death, taking the baby back to his mother to hold, to hug, and to stroke before giving him up forever.

If things progress normally, the midwife will "catch" the baby, put it right up on the mother's abdomen, and try to sit with her awhile, awaiting the placenta's delivery, assisting with breast-feeding instruction before leaving them alone.

Again, Kay keeps the mother informed of whatever is happening—when the baby is weighed and footprinted, when Apgar scores for newborn development are assessed, when drops are instilled into the eyes.

During the postpartum phase, Kay returns for more teaching, reinforcing previous information and introducing new concerns. She tries to give the patient options about discharge. Some leave as soon as six to twelve hours. Most stay twenty-four to thirty-six hours. But, all things being equal, there is the option. She reassures the mother that she should call if things get too burdensome or if she feels unusually blue or depressed.

Instead of the usual posthospitalization six-week stretch, Kay always sets up the first visit after two weeks. These are crucial weeks, particularly for a first birth, when a woman's body and life-style have been so changed and a new person is in her home. There is so much to adjust to.

When they need her, Kay wants her patients to know she is there.

13

"Different Responsibilities"

Nurse Practitioners

The certified nurse practitioner (CNP) movement started in the 1960s. The concept allowed for nurses with extra education to work jointly with a physician, handling the less difficult cases. It was hoped this would expand health care to underserved rural and inner-city populations. Being a CNP also allowed nurses the option of professional advancement without having to abandon patient contact for the more conventional route into education or administrative functions.

Joyce was a junior in college during the late 1960s. She was drawn to the idea of a nursing practice with expanded authority and autonomy, and she believed it would be her nursing niche. She did staff nursing for a few years before returning to graduate school for her master's degree as an adult family nurse practitioner.

She was one of the first to enter independent practice. It was still quite revolutionary in the mid-seventies. She was hired to develop a freestanding clinic in the largest city in a northeastern state. A local corporation helped underwrite the project. It was to function as an extension of a university school of nursing providing graduate-level clinical rotations as well as serving an underprivileged population.

The position was wonderful, a model of collaborative practice in health care. Joyce worked with a physician fifteen hours each week. He stopped in each morning to make sure things were going smoothly, but she saw most of the patients.

It soon became apparent that many of the key political players in the state's health game had not been consulted in the formation of the clinic. When the project went into effect, all hell broke loose. There was no trouble when practitioners were taking care of people on Indian reservations or in remote areas, but step into the city . . .

The state medical association became threatened and went to work on the clinic's physician, pressuring him to leave, questioning the legality of his supervision of Joyce's practice. Then they went to work on the subsidizing corporation. They even implied that they would bring suit for practicing medicine without a license.

It was about the toughest fifteen months of Joyce's life. Eventually, the project was phased down, her practice taken over by a physician. It was a concept ahead of its time. Joyce moved into nursing education.

Today, nurse practitioners practice as primary care givers in all fifty states. There are several thousand in New York State alone. They are employed by hospitals, outpatient clinics, and in private-practice settings. Depending upon location, varying degrees of independence of practice exist. In many states, nurse practitioners diagnose illness and order medication regimes and therapeutic interventions. A 1986 Office of Technology Assessment study reported that CNPs "provide care that is equivalent in quality to the care provided by physicians for similar problems."

K. C. is a tallish, rangy woman with long brunette hair. In 1977, she was traveling in Europe, needing to do something different with her life. She already possessed a bachelor's degree in psychology and had done some counseling work for the state. Still, she had found no direction in her life. She concluded she wanted to be in a service industry that had a lot of contact with people.

Her personality demanded that there also be some sort of informational or academic challenge involved.

She had done some volunteer work in a clinic and became interested in going to medical school. She saw how there could be some fun to medicine, in the detective work involved, the processing of information toward a diagnosis. At Michigan State, she told an interview committee what she really wanted to do in medicine, and she was told, "You don't want to be a doctor. You want to be a nurse."

She was taken aback, but, through talking with nurses, she realized that, philosophically, she *didn't* want to be a doctor—she wanted to be a nurse.

"I wouldn't have made it as a doctor. I don't have that obsessive compulsiveness that you need to be a good one, that computer type of brain. That and a good heart. Most doctors don't have the heart. It's tough to have both. I think I'm more intuitive than I am organized. Plus, I was older when I went back to nurse practitioner school. I was twenty-nine when I started, and I wasn't willing to sacrifice that kind of time from my life.

"I think I'm almost a genuinely nice person—not quite, but almost—and I think I wanted to contribute that to health care."

She was accepted into Yale's three-year, master's-level nurse practitioner program and graduated as an adult family nurse practitioner.

Her first position was in an overcrowded metropolitan city jail, one of the largest in the country. There were over two thousand men and three hundred women. She went primarily because she wanted to work someplace where she would see many patients and have a lot of diversity. The salary was adequate, but what was really attractive was the prospect of unlimited overtime. Her Yale loan commitment was tremendous.

She was placed in charge of the women's division. Everyone who arrived had to have a physical performed within twenty-four hours. She hadn't done a GYN exam in two years, and then only one. Most of it was conveyer-belt care, but she got diversity—hepatitis, AIDS, pneumonia, drug and alcohol withdrawal, teenagers pregnant with their third or fourth child, suicide attempts, VD.

She only had one acutely harrowing experience. It concerned a young man who had just been sentenced to five years. Usually when sentenced to do time in excess of a year, prisoners were immediately transported to the penitentiary. This guy complained of an ailment, though, and was returned to the dispensary. He was very upset about his sentence and wanted to hurt someone, break something. He lost control.

"You can yell all you want, bitch," he raved, tearing at her. "They can shoot me, and I don't care."

She had a heavy door in her office that she rarely closed. He tried to barricade it against the officers. But because he couldn't man the barricade *and* assault her simultaneously, they were able to break through before any real harm was done.

Taking social histories from prisoners, trying to find a coherent line and follow it through the complexity and chaos of the person's life, was particularly difficult. There was little chance to be introspective. Administrative support was also often less than optimal.

"I was working ten- and twelve-hour days, fighting constantly for enough supplies, better staffing, and new equipment. I was constantly getting flak for sending people out to the hospital—I mean, we had asthmatics who weren't responding to our little Bronkosol treatments, and we weren't able to hang an aminophylline drip.

"Then two things made me reevaluate my decision to work there. First, I was told not to do any more PAP smears on anyone—and for many of these women, this was the only place they'd ever had a PAP test—and then I was told I'd only be getting regular-sized specula. (Apparently the company that ran the medical department—this was a private concern

from another state—had underbid in its attempt to gain the
city contract.) Now, even if some of these women hadn't been
arrested for prostitution, most of them had multiple sexual
partners. The thought of a single-sized speculum made me
cringe.''

She stayed just shy of a year, then left to take a position within
a sprawling university health care system. It's a clinic for employees and HMO members, very different from the prison. She
has her own office with a desk and prints on the wall. There is
carpet on the floor. It's clean, and people never seem to curse
at her anymore. Sometimes it gets a little boring, but it's also
nice to have patients who can verbalize concerns.

It is an outpatient ambulatory clinic treating a broad spectrum
of illnesses. K. C. has her own patient pool. She has diagnosed
the gamut, from colds and sore throats to non-symptomatic HIV
and cancer, from diabetes and hypertension to blood dyscrasias
and cardiac insufficiency.

Diagnosing can be very problematic. She has had people come
to see her, people in their sixties and seventies who were feeling
just fine, only to find out they had cancer. Recently, K. C. has
been dealing with a situation in which an older woman, Estelle,
came in for a walk-in visit. She seemed to have bronchitis.
K. C. ordered a routine chest film, mostly because she would
be seeing her again in a few weeks for a checkup anyway.

The film returned positive for a high probability of cancer.

Because she didn't know the radiologist who did the original
read, K. C. took the film to the chief of radiology for another
opinion. He gave a very dramatic presentation.

''I think this is metastasis,'' he said, his hand tracing the
snowfall effect on the film. ''You've got to find the site of ori-
gin.''

This woman was going to be coming in for a routine H & P.
K. C. consulted with her senior CNP. Should she tell the lady
her CXR was abnormal? If not, how much should she tell?

"Just tell her, 'This is an abnormality. We need to look into it. Now I need to ask you a lot of detailed questions.' "

When Estelle arrived, K. C. sat beside her on a stool. As soon as she began to speak, Estelle gripped her knee. She knew exactly what was being said. They stared at each other. K. C.'s stomach flipped and her mouth dried up. She reached down and held Estelle's arm, her hand still gripping K. C.'s knee, trembling. Neither spoke for a long time.

Such circumstances—K. C. didn't *have* to get that X ray. Estelle had simply complained of a cough. Her lungs sounded okay. There was no pain. She's sixty-seven.

"She's a wonderful lady. She has a great deal of grace. I've found with her, more than with anyone else, that I sometimes almost want to cry as we're sitting there. She's come to see me as things have gone on. She's connected with a pulmonary specialist here. He talks to me when he does his office visits. Her husband's also recently been diagnosed with CA and is having radiation treatments.

"She'll come in basically to talk, get some Librium to get her by. I see her, and I just want to hug her. She's going in the hospital this weekend for her biopsy, and I'm going to go up and visit her. I've never done that before. I feel very strongly that I don't want to get emotionally involved with any of my patients, but, for whatever reason, I think this will be okay. It's an intuitive sense I've learned to trust.

"I think I'm a chauvinist in that I expect more of women than I do of men. I like the way women relate more than men. I'm heterosexual. I have a man I'm deeply in love with. I have male friends. But I think in the psychological evolution of the sexes, that women got a better shake than men. It's easy to be rational—all you have to do is sit down and think, going from A to B to C. It's tougher to be intuitive, to be verbal and articulate about things that aren't real in the sense of being measurable."

Anna has been a CNP since 1985, employed at a medium-sized general hospital in Maryland. Her schedule allows her a variety of experiences, something she likes. CNPs at her hospital rotate every two months between five different services—medical patients, preadmission testing, telemetry, private physicians' patients, and a surgical rotation. There is the possibility of a sixth rotation being added, meaning she would spend only two months of any given year in one place. That variety makes for an interesting mix, reducing work stress considerably.

The hospital is under contract to staff the city's VD clinics. Nurse practitioners take turns, and Monday morning is Anna's.

It is her job to diagnose and manage acute ailments. They try to provide clients with anonymity. Each client is given a number at the reception desk, and then sit until it is called. Inside her office, it's all very straightforward. Anna takes a history and performs a physical. If it's a man, a simple genital test with urethral smear will suffice; obtain a gram stain and evaluate the pathogen.

Usually it's gonorrhea, chlamydia, or herpes. Occasionally it's the stigmata of syphilis, requiring a more elaborate, epidemiological workup. The CDC estimates that between eight and ten million Americans at any given time are infected with a sexually transmitted disease (STD). Anna prescribes meds and arranges for a follow-up test for cure. She also provides referral cards for partners. Sometimes people actually show up with those cards.

AIDS information is a major thrust of the clinic, to raise the general knowledge level. Anna and her co-workers find little change in the sex habits of the mostly young, black, heterosexual population they serve. There continues to be a widespread belief that because they are not gay, they won't get it. Posters quoting Louis Sullivan, secretary of Health and Human Services, his photo affixed, cover the walls of the waiting room: "It appears that the (center) of the AIDS epidemic is shifting into lower-income, minority neighborhoods, where drug abuse drives its spread.'' More recently, pictures of Magic Johnson have been added.

Anna does a lot of teaching about how STDs are spread and how they can be avoided, clearing up some myths about ineffective preventive practices. Women still believe that douching helps, when in actuality it can drive the infection further north. Some think they have immunity because they've had it before, like it's measles. Some believe they can tell by personal appearance if a person is diseased or not.

The clinic is in a dangerous part of town. Men are especially interested in the lady who ''burned'' them. Anna is diagnosing venereal disease to people who know they didn't *get* it. They're pissed at whoever *gave* it to them, and intend to get even. They're going to put a fist in a face, a boot up a butt. The potential for violence is there, and it has occurred. People have been shot dead for unfaithfulness right in the waiting room.

It is in the waiting room that most problems occur, usually among groups of young men who are acting out anxiety, stirring the broth, getting loud or a little too clever, hitting a raw nerve. The shoving and cursing start. A police officer is assigned to each clinic. Anna sometimes has to call the clinic cop to sit in the room.

Once clients enter the office, one on one, things pretty much settle down. Anna gives them a thumbnail sketch of anatomy and physiology, telling the men that their partner may not even know she is infected because of the way she is built. Many of the clients had this information somewhere along the line, in junior high, but everybody was goofing off, ''woo-wooing,'' and hooting, and they didn't pick it up correctly. Most are very amenable to whatever instruction Anna gives them.

It's an interesting rotation, despite the fact that most people tend to grimace and give her a long-distance stare, inching perceptibly away when she tells them about it. But, basically, the clients are healthy young people who are quite troubled that they have contracted a venereal disease. The worst part is when there is an infected child, ten or eleven, who doesn't know what happened to her. Usually she will be accompanied by her mother. It can become very delicate, teasing out information, deciding whether or not to phone Child Protective Services.

It's much easier having some streetwise kid who is in for the fifth time in six months. After a while Anna started to appreciate such guys.

"So, tell me what I told you the last time," she can say when doing the educational part. "Run it by me. . . ."

Because she loses half the day, Mondays often make for major hassles. At the hospital, she must quickly round on her patients, checking lab results and getting a brief report of how each one's weekend went. There is also usually at least one admission awaiting workup. Over time, Anna learned which corners she could safely trim.

Orthopedics, her current rotation, is a surgical service. Arthroplasty, joint reconstruction, is its speciality. There are between twenty-five and thirty-five patients on the service. Many are in and out of the hospital rather rapidly. Patients who are admitted because of traumas, like fingers or limbs torn off or so mangled they can't be reimplanted, necessitating a clean amputation, are usually young and otherwise healthy, and have particularly brief admissions.

Hip replacements are one of the major surgical specialities offered by the hospital. Some patients even refer to it as "the hip hospital." Hips are usually a ten-day to two-week admission. The patients are frequently over seventy years old—or look it—and plagued by chronic conditions affecting their ability to heal. They are where Anna focuses most of her attention. Normally they are hypertensive or diabetic, or have something else that will tend to be overlooked by the surgical team, who concentrate on whatever joint it is they are replacing.

Surgeons are famous for not wanting to deal with the fact that a patient is diabetic. The condition of the surgical wound is about the extent of their concern. If it looks good, life is good. The rest is a sort of black box. Surgical services just want the patient *out*, yesterday.

Anna keeps a running profile on each patient's medical history, what pre-surgical meds they were on, what therapies they were utilizing, and monitors them for any resurgence of preexisting conditions. If someone's diabetes is severe, her contribution is to get a medical consult to manage it. If it is stable, she will simply institute what she thinks is an appropriate sliding scale of insulin.

Nurse practitioners take admissions in random turns, following each patient throughout their stay, doing the H & P, writing admission orders, and consulting with the physician about further testing when results return. Today Anna had two admissions waiting when she arrived. The first was somewhat unusual: an Asian woman in her mid-thirties who came in with a diagnosis of vascular necrosis. Basically, her joints are self-destructing, the blood supply having died due to steroids she was given for her asthma as a child. She has already had one major joint replaced, but the hardware has broken down. She's in to see if it is possible to have it screwed tight again.

The second admission is more the norm: a Caucasian male in for knee surgery. Synovectomy is the removal of the synovial membrane, which lines joint capsules in an attempt to forestall the progression of rheumatoid arthritis. It is obvious to Anna upon entering his room that Stanley H. has multiple other medical problems as well. His shortness of breath and repeated coughs indicate a chronic respiratory problem, probably bronchitis. He has the obese build and dusky, almost cyanotic, skin coloring that go along with the disease. The slang for such people is "a blue bloater." He is hypertensive.

The history part of Mr. H.'s H & P confirms what Anna had guessed. At fifty-six, he is a chronic smoker, two to four packs a day, a frequent beer imbiber, and consumer of fast foods, laden in fats, starches, and salt. Typical of those with the illness, which progresses "silently" for years before symptoms fully blossom, Stanley has sought no medical consultation for his transient discomforts. Anna writes orders for several diagnostic tests: arterial blood gases, chest X rays, and spirometry.

Upon questioning, Stanley displays little insight into how his personal practices are contributing to his own demise. More disheartening, he shows little inclination to change his behavior. When Anna suggests an exercise and abstinence regime, Stanley scoffs.

"Doc's gonna fix it all up for me. Says he'll take some fluid out of my knees to avoid the arthritis, and the pain should stop."

"The membrane is removed." Anna sketches a quick representation of a knee joint, supplying him with more information about the procedure. "But that's not a cure, Mr. H. The membrane will grow back, and the disease might well resurface. But you could certainly have a better chance of not having pain recur if your knees weren't carrying around excess weight."

"Uh-huh," he responds dismissively. "We'll see, okay?"

Anna asks if excess sputum production, a common symptom of bronchitis, is a problem.

"Yeah, as a matter of fact, it is," he says, adding in the American mode, "Is there something I can take for that?"

Anna continues to find the illness orientation of health care demoralizing. The desire to place emphasis on the preventive end of the health care spectrum is a philosophy that predates Florence Nightingale. But illness is still what is stressed in nursing and medicine. Illness is where insurance money is.

She understands the allure of technology. Laser surgery and baboon hearts in babies are amazing. Plus, they garner headlines and careers are made, funding following flashiness. It's a lot less glamorous to work with obese people to change their unhealthy dietary habits. Or to get people to stop smoking so they don't trash out their lungs. Or to bolster someone's ability to manage stress so they don't become riddled with peptic ulcers or meet the stress with heavy drinking and drugs.

It's very simple, unglamorous, un*profit*able work, but it accounts for so much of what happens to people who land in hospital beds needing her care, a physician's care, and a respiratory therapist's care.

"It frustrates me that people who were born with healthy bodies abuse them. I think that probably has political ramifications, social ramifications. The life-style in this country is very unhealthy, harried, consumptive, and excessive. There's so much attention to comfort, some to the mind, and very little to the spirit. We pay the price in our health."

Anna enjoys being able to order her own day, not being bound to a particular floor, being a troubleshooter. She can be in different places in one day, on different floors seeing different patients. Practitioners visit each one of their patients on a daily basis, writing progress notes, following labs, and reading their X rays or getting them read.

Her inpatient caseload varies, from day to day and from service to service, divided among four practitioners. If somebody is off for a day, it rises proportionately. On a weekend, Anna covers the entire census: there are thirty-plus fairly complex medical problems to watch and take action on if needed.

Sometimes elderly persons whose workup is done—their hip mended or pneumonia resolved—can't be discharged because of a social problem, such as being too frail to return home. Because of their financial situation, it is difficult to find a nursing home to take them. So they stay, day after day. The hospital will probably wind up eating most of the cost, but what Anna finds distressing is the knowledge that if they stay long enough, they are sure to get sick. There are so many bugs in hospitals. They'll end up with a uterine-track infection or a wound infection, or fall out of bed and fracture the new hip or a bone of older vintage. It is awful to see someone languishing in pain and disease because they were in a hospital.

Little of what she does on a regular basis bears much resemblance to what she was taught in her master's-level practitioner program. The focus of her education was to prepare her to handle ambulatory patients in a clinic setting. The only time she spent in a hospital was when she was learning to do a history and physical. Once she was through the mechanics of performing a physical exam from start to finish, everything else was in a clinic.

Suddenly, she was writing prescriptions. When she started, she didn't even know how to order IVs for people, how much they should get, how fast the infusion rate. For a while, she would simply order up another brew of what they had before. Then she talked to other practitioners and a few physicians, and figured it out, memorizing the thirty or so drugs used most often, concentrating on the prototypes. Those thirty drugs got her a long way down the road.

When she shows up on a floor, Anna believes she is seen as a solver of problems for the staff nurses. Unlike residents who won't answer their pages, when beeped, Anna appears. And she is authorized to do useful things. If somebody's IV is running out and he needs another liter, she can write for that. If somebody's having chest pain and turning blue, she can do what needs to be done in the first few minutes when the nurses are getting things rolling, like authorizing tests the staff know will be needed so that when the doc does show up, the process is that much farther along.

Periodically, when there's no other pair of hands around, Anna helps out with rolling a patient over or transferring to a stretcher, not disdaining the kind of work floor nurses do or making labor distinctions. Med-surg nursing is one of the most draining jobs in the world anybody can do. Anna has done it herself and respects what is required.

There are days, however, when there simply aren't enough hours, when she'll say to a patient, "I'll put you on the bedpan; please ring for your nurse when you're ready to get off."

It is rare for Anna to differ with the diagnosis made by physicians. There was an instance when a patient had a swollen leg. He was being treated for syphilis. Anna was doubtful, believing the problem to be an occult abscess. She set about establishing this by employing a low-level assessment technique, taking measurements of the girth of his thigh. She marked each measurement with a ballpoint pen, demonstrating that it was growing larger.

Because something concrete was established, her opinion gained validity. The physician pursued it. He performed an ultrasound, and the abscess was seen. In his case, he was appreciative where another physician might have resented her. Nobody likes to be wrong, particularly in his own area of expertise. But, as a result of this experience, Anna believes that she and the physician feel more respectful of each other.

Anna has great concerns about the state of the nursing profession. She hears a lot from patients about the often negative quality of nursing care they receive. Unless it is something dangerous, it goes no farther than to Anna. She doesn't think reporting individual nurses will make a difference. Most hospitals are bending over backward to keep the nurses they have, regardless of quality.

She thinks there are a lot of nurses who would normally do adequate work who aren't because of current conditions. There are all these buzzwords and catchphrases around—DRG high acuity, nursing shortage, overwork, underpaid, burnout. What they add up to is a general slipping of the level that everybody should be shooting for. Part of it may be beyond nursing, the reflection of a more general breakdown, the way people are brought up these days, the casual crumbling of social structures, the behavior accepted from public figures.

"There have always been nurses with high professional standards who went that forty-seventh mile to try and do it all. But I think there are a lot of cruisers out there, and now, with the shortage, is the perfect time to excuse less than adequate behavior.

"There will always be people who will try to do more than they can, just because it's in them to do so. I hope there are enough of them."

When accepting this assignment, her first as a new practitioner, Anna budgeted it out for two years. The first year would be spent on learning. She assumed it would take at least that long to finish her education, to be able to pull her own weight. The second year would be for giving back, being of some use to the hospital. She is comfortable with what she does now. That first year she was so incredibly anxious.

The hardest adaptation to nursing practice for Anna has been to maintain a high degree of efficiency and focused concentration in the performance of repetitive tasks. By nature, she tends to ruminate, to think things through. It has been a hard discipline, both as a staff nurse and now as a CNP, to keep rolling, to go from one task to the next without pause for reflection or to make any kind of meaning out of anything she is doing on a daily basis.

Anna has since completed the apprenticeship she contracted with herself and feels at liberty to seek whatever kind of speciality she desires. What that is has not yet become clear. She doesn't know where she could find a position with more variety than what is available here. But she is not sure she can stomach staying put till the end of her days doing useful adjunctive types of things. The next logical step is to become a more independent kind of practitioner, like in an HMO.

"I keep coming back to the fact that I'd rather be helping someone grow than dealing with the consequences of unhealthy behavior. At some point, hopefully, that's all going to come together, and I'll recognize the next step. Then I can shed the next layer of skin in growth."

14

"The Nature of the Work"

Teaching

JoAnn removes her lab coat, the only article of clothing that could identify her as being in health care, and sits behind her desk. In conservative dress and jewelry, her hair pulled back smartly into a bun, she could be thought an attorney, a banker, or a stockbroker as easily as the university professor she is.

In the hallway, workmen pound and pry, carry file cabinets to the elevator, disassemble desks and bookcases, roll up the rugs. They are subdividing a conference room to create office space for two part-time teachers hired by the school of nursing. It was just a few years ago, as part of the nursing shortage ripple effect, that the entire school's offices were moved across campus. With enrollments on the decline, smaller quarters seemed indicated. Now, with applications rebounding, there has been talk of moving the school once again, but everyone is taking a wait-and-see attitude, realizing the entire health care field is in too great a state of flux to make such plans.

JoAnn has learned to hedge all bets when predicting the future of her profession. Her own office reflects the disarray of pending relocation. Her texts and periodicals have either been boxed or sit in stacks awaiting crating. Somewhere in there she has several reports by the Department of Health and Human Services with predictions about the future of the

.....sing needs. One, from the mid-eighties, pre-
.....t by 1990 the number of RNs available to work
..... exceed the need for them by 40,000. A second re-
.....t—this one from 1990—stated that at that time, there was
an actual shortfall of almost 200,000 RNs and that these
numbers, even by conservative estimate, could climb into
the mid-300,000s by the end of the century.

All this talk about what will and won't be the case by the
end of the nineties leaves JoAnn a little bemused. At the
beginning of the eighties, very few people had even heard of
AIDS, pharmacology textbooks were teaching that cocaine
was nonaddictive, what few ''homeless'' could be found were
called derelicts, and it was common for patients with physical
ills to stay in hospitals for months and psychiatric patients for
years.

Today she only wonders if whatever the nineties have in store
will be able to surprise her. And she hopes it won't leave her so
numbed that she doesn't care.

JoAnn began teaching within a couple of years of completing
her master's degree. Earlier in her career, she'd worked for a
public health department in another part of the country. She
found the part of the job that she most enjoyed was the teaching
she did. Drawn to a Sunbelt state, she took a full-time post at a
university nursing school, eventually earning her Ph.D.

''I thoroughly enjoyed doctoral study. I enjoyed the course
work. I came to it not knowing anything about adult development, the stages of adulthood, career counseling techniques—any of it. It was something that I was and still am
profoundly interested in.''

In addition to the teaching, she enjoys performing research
and practice, though she is quick to note that she hasn't been
''practicing'' nursing for over a decade. The only patient contact she has today is through supervision of graduate-level

nursing students. She is the first to admit she is not out there in the trenches, and considers herself no more representative of the typical nurse than the guy who runs the subway. She has four times the education of the average nurse and doesn't deal at the same socioeconomic level anymore. She is just not there.

What she finds disturbing is meeting colleagues who are not even aware that they're not there. She knows doctorally prepared nurses who really believe that they represent nurses and nursing. From her perspective, somewhere along the line nursing became terribly academic, where academia became the yardstick for measuring success within the profession, fueling the entry-level feud that continues to smolder and flare. Being an educator, she recognizes that for a profession to survive and flourish, it requires an ivory tower as much as a front line.

"The ivory tower, though, should exist to enhance and assist the front line, which is the true work of the profession. In national nursing leadership circles, however, I've witnessed an attitude that the front line has become synonymous with ineptitude, in that if a nurse is not clever enough to get out of direct patient care, she must be slow-witted or unmotivated."

She has no doubt that nursing has made tremendous strides forward in the last fifty years, especially in terms of shaking to the roots the whole militaristic, religious heritage of diploma schools. The subsequent disruption has contributed to nursing's present crisis, but then, growth is hard. She only hopes that something just as insidiously rigid hasn't been substituted.

"Professional organizations are most important, particularly in the early stages of a profession. Unfortunately, some people become 'professional groupies.' You have your ANA [American Nurses' Association] groupie-types whose entire

...ng on this committee or that committee. It be-
...orce in and of itself, providing a sense of status and
...orth that practicing nursing does not. Their perspective
...comes highly colored and questionable in terms of where
they steer the profession.''

JoAnn has never considered nursing anything other than a
profession. It's not a job, but something to which she has
committed herself. She has invested two decades of her life
moving upward within the profession, having made the correct career decisions—BSN, MSN, Ph.D.—and feels a vested
interest in its survival. However, she harbors grave concerns
about that very issue. She has a horrible aching vision of
nursing becoming nothing but a footnote in the annals of
medical history.

To keep current within the field, she deals with nurses at all
levels, from the bedside to the boardroom. In addition to floor
nurse contacts she made while supervising students in clinical
rotations, she also does a fair amount of consultation in hospitals
around the country and feels very much in touch with the beat
of the profession.

Most recently, she has been working with a lot of hospital
nursing professional development (PD) coordinators. PD coordinators are often master's-prepared clinical specialists who work
to enhance staff functioning, orienting new employees and
keeping staff nurses current with in-service lectures for specific
practice problems. JoAnn consistently hears from these people
about feeling terribly stretched, overwhelmed by circumstances
created by the shortage and DRGs, crack and AIDS and under-
funding. Hospitals are hemorrhaging funds at terrific rates. Some
are happy to receive Medicare reimbursement of a dime on a
dollar.

Usually, when things get bad in hospitals, PD personnel
are the first nurses to get trimmed. They're just not frontline
people. Those who have managed to hang on tell their stories
about their frustrations as ''developers of professional peo-

ple,'' when in reality—between the increased use of agency nurses and the staggering staff turnover rates—all they have time to do is orient new people. The old concept of coordinators acting as "patient advocates" and "patient educators"—all the umbrella duties they once performed—has been tossed out the window. It frightens JoAnn as a nurse, an educator, and as a health consumer.

As an academic, she has witnessed the overall trend in the profession: because fewer young women were entering the field at the close of the 1980s, nursing schools—in order to stay afloat financially—were being forced to accept less qualified candidates who require remediation into programs with the hope that they can be molded into competent practitioners. The impact of the recession and the continued growth in health care careers have sparked growing enrollments in nursing schools. However, because of the reduction in faculties in the previous five years, many students needed to be turned away. The National League of Nursing estimated that in 1990 almost 5 percent of full-time teaching positions were vacant. A survey by the American Association of Colleges of Nursing cited seventy-eight institutions turning down as many as 2,652 qualified applicants. From an economic standpoint, it's hard to see this problem changing soon. In 1991, a nurse with a two-year associate degree could earn almost a thousand dollars more as a staff nurse than a doctorally prepared nursing instructor.

A good deal of JoAnn's time is spent counseling nursing graduate-school candidates. The decision to enter nursing grad school is a tough one. She talks with many women and men, generally in their early thirties, who are questioning their choice of career. From where she sits, she watches some of the best and brightest leaving the profession at mid-life. Some are going into law school or business administration, deciding to play the game from a corporate standpoint, and doing very well financially. Some are going into medicine. Some are just going.

She constantly feels the pang of moral dilemma when dealing

helping them make decisions about their fu-
to deal with her own feelings about the issue:
can, in all honesty, continue to encourage bright,
nurses to go into nursing. It often feels self-serving
to encourage them, because that's what pays her salary. She
tends to present other options to them: "Are you certain you
don't want to go to medical school? What is it about nursing
that makes you want to stay?"

She spent much of her morning today conferring with a young
woman named Annalisa, who is considering going on for graduate study in clinical nursing. Annalisa's husband was doing
well financially, affording her the option of returning to school.
She was someone who was young enough to explore other options, while old enough to remember the last shortage. At that
time, there was a lot of talk about improving the environment
for nursing practice, enhancement of professional standing, and
according authority to complement responsibility. In the long
run, though, not much changed. She pondered what amount of
her time and energy—and a questionable number of thousands
of dollars—she wanted to invest in a profession in such dire
straights.

JoAnn perceives a problem for nurses that goes beyond the
health care system to the very social agenda of the nation. Quite
simply, it is difficult to demand and then receive respect for
doing something that society itself takes for granted. Though
she rarely mentions the analogy between nursing and mother-
hood—knowing it makes people livid—she believes there are
corollaries.

"It's like when women say, 'Put a price on housework.
What would it cost you to run a household without me?' It's
estimated somewhere near fifty thousand dollars a year for
running and maintaining a home, raising children, and doing
all the nurturing wifely and motherly things. Not to mention
the logistics of shopping, transportation, paying bills, etc. All
the vague, desultory tasks that comprise a life."

But the system only appreciates what it can quantify, tasks reduced to a dollar sign. There is no profit attached to empathy, interpersonal contact, encouragement, and caring. The system does not value what nurses do best, which is helping someone heal through adversity or die with dignity. It is hard to put a dollar sign on "caring." But just ask anyone who has ever felt terrified and abandoned what value it held to have another human being be there with them on what Susan Sontag calls the "nightside of life."

And being there is the whole point of nursing.

Along with Annalisa's other professional concerns, she was quite worried about AIDS; aside from her husband, she also had two small children to care for. She wanted to know if JoAnn was personally afraid of taking care of AIDS patients.

JoAnn thought it an interesting question, coming from a candidate for graduate study in a health profession.

"I couldn't help but be struck by the irony of it, how it reflected the point we have come to—in health care in general and nursing in particular. I tend to look at things from a historical, broader perspective, and it struck me that one of the ironies of the whole AIDS crisis is in context of the last twenty years, when we've had our noses buried in technologies and advancements in physiological monitoring—intensive care units coming out the wazoo, this kind of catheter, that type of machine—and our whole attitude of: 'We're gonna solve it all!'

"But now it looks like we're going to go out of this century the same way we came in—people dying in vast numbers from infectious diseases.

"I can't help but see the irony in terms of the role of nursing, historically, as far as infection control and the managing of sick and dying people is concerned. Those of us— particularly at my level in the profession—who are advocates of the care of the well, with preventive practices and health pro-

...ssed as the key role of the nurse, can see ...ne greatest demand now, and for the foresee- ...will be the compassionate care of the sick and

...which is exactly how nursing got started.''

About the Author

Michael Brown graduated from nursing school at Hahnemann University in 1983. Prior to that he worked as a psychiatric technician in the nursing departments of several hospitals. Since 1990 he has been on the staff of Johns Hopkins Hospital. He currently lives in Baltimore, Maryland, with his wife, Melody Simmons, a journalist, and their daughter.